RADICAL RELIEF

A Guide to Overcome Chronic Pain

Return to a full, active life using pain science, mindfulness, and Acceptance and Commitment Therapy

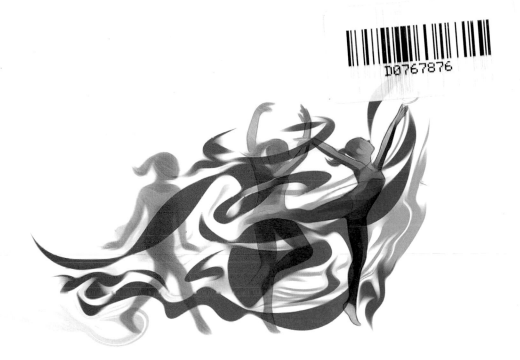

Joe Tatta, PT, DPT, CNS

© 2020 Joe Tatta, PT, DPT, CNS

Published by OPTP
3800 Annapolis Lane N, Suite 165
Minneapolis, MN 55447
OPTP.com

Printed in the United States of America

Design: OPTP
Copyediting: OPTP
Illustrations: Marty Harris Illustration

The information contained herein is not intended to be a substitute for professional medical advice, diagnosis or treatment in any manner. Always seek the advice of your physician or other qualified healthcare provider with any questions you may have regarding any medical condition or before engaging in any physical fitness plan. Neither the author nor the publisher shall be liable or responsible for any loss, injury, or damage allegedly arising from any information or suggestion in this publication.

ISBN: 978-1-942-798-22-4

TABLE OF CONTENTS

PART IV
Fully Present and Aware: Be in the Moment and Relate Differently

PART V
Take Action and Do What Matters: Commit to a New and Vital Life Course

CONCLUSION

Dedication

For mom and dad, Dorothy and Anthony, for your never-ending love, acceptance, and kindness. And for my husband, Jeorge, who teaches me how to hold the tension in life lightly.

Acknowledgments

The idea for this book developed shortly after my first self-help book, *Heal Your Pain Now*, became popular in 2016. People wanted to know more about the brain and how to use the wonders of the human mind to overcome pain and live a more vital life. Mindfulness and Acceptance and Commitment Therapy were mentioned briefly but rightly deserved their own time in the sun. Radical Relief is the natural extension from that first book and is for those who have tried everything to eliminate pain but are still suffering.

Thank you to the many practitioners and colleagues who keep me growing and for the work you do each and every day to help people overcome pain. I hope this book serves as a valuable resource to enhance your practice, professional development, and to improve pain care. I also want to extend my appreciation to Cathy Lindvall and Ryan Bussman at OPTP for believing in the topic and in me and to Amy Bowman for her incredible editorial skill and support, which transformed this project. And to the many ACT practitioners and researchers who continually develop this flexible and evidence-based approach to treating pain and suffering. Finally, to the countless people living with pain, your courage and wisdom help us all grow.

Free Resources and Online Training

I have created the following resources for you to use and share with your friends and colleagues.

Website: www.integrativepainscienceinstitute.com

ACT for Chronic Pain Training: www.integrativepainscienceinstitute.com/act/

Mindfulness-Based Pain Relief Training:
www.integrativepainscienceinstitute.com/mindfulness

RELIEF: an online mindfulness community for pain care.
www.integrativepainscienceinstitute.com/relief

Book: *Heal Your Pain Now: The Revolutionary Program to Reset Your Brain and Body for a Pain-Free Life. Da Capo Press*

INTRODUCTION:
A NEW BEGINNING FOR PEOPLE LIVING WITH PAIN

If you picked up this book, there is a good chance you are experiencing long-term chronic pain. The pain may be in your back, hip, knee, neck or all over your body and may swell to a level 6, 7, 8, 9 or 10, rarely retreating long enough for you to remember what life was like before the pain. It's likely that conventional treatments haven't worked very well. In addition to costing money, pain treatments can affect mood, sleep, energy, relationships, family life and work life, and rarely provide long-term relief. Pain can erode your quality of life by stopping you from doing the things you love and being the person you were meant to be. If this is the case, you are not alone. Globally, it is estimated that about one in five, or about 1.5 billion people, suffer from chronic pain.

Acute pain is different. It typically lasts less than six months and serves an important purpose—it keeps you safe from harm. But chronic pain is something altogether different. It stays with you. Over time, chronic pain tugs and pulls you away from life. In addition to affecting relationships, family and work life, and the ability to enjoy your favorite activities, chronic pain can leave you feeling scared, anxious, sad and angry. You may find yourself struggling to control the pain and the unpleasant thoughts and emotions that go along with it. The struggle to control pain can rob you of your freedom and cause you to suffer. But it doesn't have to be this way.

There are ways to overcome and break free from chronic pain. This book contains some radical ideas ripe to change your life. Most popular pain treatments, like exercise and manual therapy, focus on treating the body—yet, science has proven that these treatments also impact how we think and how we relate to pain. The mind is affected by pain treatments, and there is no denying the role the mind plays in recovering from pain.

The word radical means: "Of or going to the root or origin; fundamental." Using Acceptance and Commitment Therapy, Radical Relief can help you overcome chronic pain by bringing you back to the root of pain and suffering: the mind.

Acceptance and Commitment Therapy: New Hope to Overcome Pain

Acceptance and Commitment Therapy, or "ACT," pronounced as one word, is a time-tested, science-backed approach that has helped thousands of people with a wide range of painful musculoskeletal conditions and mobility challenges. It can also help with stress, depression, anxiety, trauma and addiction. There is hope in the ACT approach. The aim of ACT is to help you live a rich, meaningful and active life while handling pain and the suffering that often accompanies it. This is achieved in three ways.

First, ACT helps you develop an awareness of the things you struggle with. This may be physical pain, but there are other unwanted parts of your experience that can influence your thoughts and emotions. Even the treatments prescribed for pain can contribute to the struggle. ACT helps you notice what's workable and helps you learn new skills to deal with painful thoughts, emotions and sensations. These skills will help you relate differently to pain, lessening the impact and influence pain has on your life.

Second, ACT helps you clarify and connect to what is most important and meaningful to you—these are your values. Values are like a compass that guide, inspire and motivate you to change by helping you rediscover what's most important to you.

Finally, ACT helps you take action and propels you forward toward life versus away from life. Once you've reconnected with who and what is most important, values-guided action can help you do what it takes on days when the seas are calm, and on days when the storm clouds roll in and pain or discomfort show up. ACT helps you accept what's out of your personal control and discover what's in your control, so you can commit to taking actions that bring joy, meaning, and vitality to your life.

How to Use this Book

Radical Relief was created with short, concise chapters and many of the chapters include one or two activities for deep learning. These activities are noted with this icon:

You can steadily work through the book and practice the activities to gain skills that will support your journey. Unlike your favorite novel, it is not recommended to read it all in one sitting. A best practice would be to read one or two chapters a day. Be intentional and set aside time to experience and immerse yourself in the activities. Morning is a wonderful time to do this, but do what works best for you.

As you progress through the book new memories will form and layer on top of old ones. A process of change will begin to take place. New thoughts and desires will come into your life and old ones may reappear. You'll gain an increased awareness of how pain impacts your body and your mind. You will also learn how to lessen the impact of your mind during times when it is unhelpful.

Some of the activities in Radical Relief will seem easy and may alleviate stress, promote a sense of calm and put you in contact with activities you enjoy. You may even notice your pain decreasing. These are all pleasant side effects, but not the main goal. It is often assumed that the way to reduce disability occurs through pain reduction. Conversely, mindfulness and acceptance approaches such as ACT propose that pain reduction is not necessary for reduced disability or a prerequisite to living fully. Instead, disability reduction occurs when responses to pain are changed. When unsuccessful struggles to control pain decrease, engagement in personally valued activities increases. The pain paradox is that identifying and engaging with the things we find personally meaningful and enriching precedes the alleviation of pain and suffering. Some exercises may seem challenging, possibly bringing up thoughts and feelings that are difficult or unpleasant. This is normal. At times, the process of overcoming pain is like navigating a ship through bad weather. Rough seas present useful teaching moments and an opportunity to practice with whatever shows up.

At times, a deep yearning for pain relief may appear or there may be a sudden urge to close the book and place it high on a shelf, out of sight and out of mind. This, too, is completely normal and natural. When this happens, you are likely facing some important stuff that will have a big impact on your life. If you ever start feeling this way, gently set the book down, sit up tall, take a few deep breaths and be with whatever is present. Experience your feelings for a few moments with gentle compassion and without any harsh judgment or evaluation. Afterward, pick the book back up and continue on your journey to Radical Relief.

There may also be times when you think, "This sure sounds like a strange approach to pain," or "I don't see how this is going to work for my specific pain problem." Thoughts like this are perfectly natural. Many people are hesitant or doubtful as they begin. Although there is no guarantee for any pain treatment, ACT has helped many people return to rich, meaningful and active lives, including people with fibromyalgia, back and neck pain, osteoarthritis, autoimmune conditions and migraines; as well as those suffering from depression, anxiety and trauma.

I could include volumes of scientific studies published by psychologists, physical therapists and occupational therapists showing the efficacy of this type of treatment, but that still wouldn't guarantee it will work. Here is what I can guarantee: If you quit trying whenever the thought, "This won't work," or "I don't get this," or "I don't like this" shows up, you'll stay stuck. So, even when negative thoughts pop up in your mind, will you be willing to continue trying anyway? Here-in lies a tipping point. A moment where it hurts more to avoid and not do something than to do it. There are always thoughts, feelings, sensations and memories going on inside us. Taking a step back and observing them, while still moving forward is what ACT is all about.

There is important information inside this book, waiting for you. If you agree to this work, Radical Relief will change you in two profound ways. First, you will learn to handle painful sensations, thoughts and emotions more effectively, so they don't hold you back. Second, you will have a safe place to come each day, to contemplate and rediscover what you want your life to stand for and be about. Radical Relief is about creating a rich, meaningful and active life worth living. You will gain insight into who you are, how your mind works, how you respond to pain and what you really want in life. What makes this approach radical is not that it is extreme, but that it brings you back to the root of what is important in life. Radical Relief does happen. Let's begin.

A GUIDE FOR PROFESSIONALS:
EMBRACING THE ACT MODEL FOR PAIN

When a person experiences pain, they will most naturally want to avoid it or stop it. Historically, the treatment of pain leveraged the idea of sufficient pain control and depended on a direct relationship between an identifiable physical injury and a person's report of symptoms. The amount of pain was expected to be perfectly proportional to the amount of tissue or bodily damage "causing" the pain. Entire protocols have been built around the tightly held belief in the biomedical treatment of pain which assumes a one-to-one relationship between pain and damage.[1] Unfortunately, this approach has not helped people with pain live vital lives. In many cases, it has further contributed to anxiety, depression, trauma, disability and suffering.[2]

Over the last century, this position was culturally reinforced by our industrialized medical-pharmaceutical system that continues to drive home the belief that pain is bad, people with pain are broken, they need to be fixed, and pain must be completely eliminated in order to achieve a sense of freedom and vitality. This is precisely where people living with pain struggle, become stuck and suffer. For too long important psychological factors were presumed to be contributors only in the rarest of cases where no identifiable pathology was present and the pain could be labeled as psychogenic.[3]

Thankfully, we have come a long way.

Pain care now openly embraces psychological, social, behavioral, and contextual factors, along with the biomedical.[4] This deep understanding leads the scientific community's march for effective pain care and informs research, education, clinical practice and patient self-management. However, a gargantuan fissure separates this evidence-based knowledge from the skills and systems requisite to effectively apply treatment and obtain the best possible outcomes. As practitioners, we can no longer ignore the interrelationship between neurobiological mechanisms and the psychological and social forces for optimizing individual patient outcomes. Life context matters and a method that takes all of this richness into account is desirable. Thanks to advances in new forms of cognitive behavioral therapy, practitioners have access to an evidence-based treatment to serve those living with pain. This treatment is Acceptance and Commitment Therapy.[5]

Psychological Flexibility as a Foundational Aspect of Pain Care

A modern exploration of human suffering suggests chronic pain isn't the enemy and that it doesn't need to be stopped, eliminated or controlled to live a rich, meaningful and active life.[6] Rather than focusing on changing physical or psychological pain directly, ACT seeks to change the function of those events and the individual's relationship to them. Supported by research in Relational Frame Theory, ACT informs us that psychological suffering is often caused by the interaction between language and cognition and its influence on human behavior.[7,8] ACT targets the underlying processes hypothesized to be involved in suffering, and its alleviation. While pain hurts, it is the psychological struggle with pain that causes humans to suffer. This makes an ACT approach to living with chronic pain altogether different and refreshing. It helps patients accept all types of unwanted and unpleasant inner experiences.

There is no need to pump the breaks or overly manage pain to live fully. In many ways, ACT works to reverse the negative consequences that many people with pain have endured for years. Attempts to control pain can sometimes cause more harm than good, both to the body and to a person's peace of mind.

ACT uses acceptance, mindfulness, commitment and behavior change strategies to improve vitality. As a process-based therapy[9], six therapeutic processes all contribute to a positive psychological skill. The six processes are acceptance, cognitive defusion, present moment awareness, self as context, values and committed action.[10]

Acceptance is the ability to actively embrace unwanted private experiences, including pain, thoughts, feelings and memories, without attempting to change their frequency or form. Acceptance is not a passive process, nor does it imply giving in to pain, resignation or tolerance. This is an active and open posture of curiosity and interest in our feelings, memories, bodily sensations and thoughts. The goal is not to reduce symptoms but to increase how we respond to the presence of these behavior narrowing experiences.

Cognitive defusion is the ability to see thoughts as what they are, not as what they say they are. Thoughts can often have a literal quality to them. Cognitive defusion and mindfulness techniques are used to create more flexibility in the presence of challenging thoughts by bringing awareness to the process of ongoing thinking.

Present moment awareness actively focuses on experiences as they are occurring now, in the moment, in real time. Attention to pain can pull you into the past or future and exacerbate rumination, catastrophizing and worry. Attention focused and mindfulness exercises are used to train a flexible present moment awareness.

Self as context or the "observer self" helps patients to notice a distinction between observed thoughts and the person who observes. This perspective provides a safe psychological space for facing painful feelings or thoughts. A self as context act is fostered by mindfulness, metaphors and perspective-taking exercises.

Values are unique to ACT. They rev up behavior change and maintain motivation. ACT encourages the clarification of cloudy values and the full exploration of personally held values. ACT uses metaphors, experiential exercises, self-exploration and writing exercises as ways to clarify values.

Committed action is about choosing a course of action guided by personally held values. ACT encourages the development of larger and larger patterns of action linked to chosen values.

These six processes can be folded into three and describe a behavior that is open, aware and active. Open includes the two processes (acceptance and cognitive defusion), Aware (present moment awareness and self as context), and Active (values and committed action). The six core processes and three components are commonly organized in what is referred to as the ACT hexaflex (see next page). These are at work throughout Radical Relief in its metaphors, stories, and exercises, although not explicitly mentioned to alleviate the reader of confusion and overly technical jargon. ACT is not a didactic or instructive approach, and avoids lengthy explanations. It is an experiential therapy and thus each chapter includes an exercise requiring contact with the body, mind and heart.

At the core of ACT is **psychological flexibility**. Psychological flexibility can be defined as contacting the present moment as a conscious human being, fully and without defense, as it is and not as it says it is and persisting or changing in behavior in the service of chosen values. All six processes are interconnected, work together and contribute to training psychological flexibility. With the development of greater psychological flexibility, even people with the most retractable pain are able to move toward better health and a rich, meaningful, and active life.[11, 12]

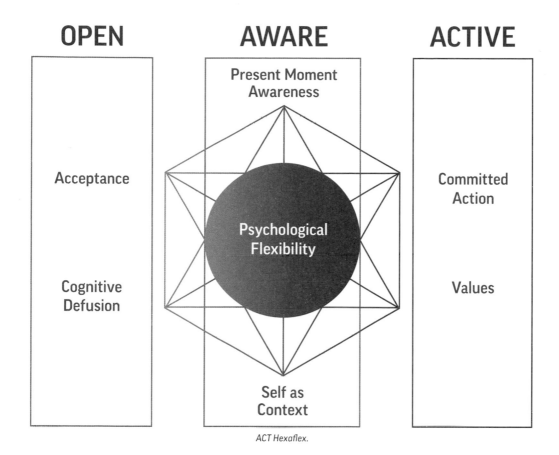

OPEN   **AWARE**   **ACTIVE**

Present Moment Awareness

Acceptance

Psychological Flexibility

Committed Action

Cognitive Defusion

Values

Self as Context

ACT Hexaflex.

How ACT Differs from Pain Education or Traditional Cognitive Behavioral Therapy

People living with pain experience many types of thoughts, feelings, memories and physical sensations. These experiences can be pleasant, unpleasant or neutral. They may influence a person to avoid, eliminate, struggle or make attempts to change them. People with pain reduce their activity, engage in excessive thoughts about pain, ruminate about the cause of pain, visit multiple practitioners, overmedicate, and find ways to distract. The ever-expanding behaviors that develop in an effort to control pain squeezes out the joy and human potential. This persistent focus on pain control narrows life and is harmful to wellbeing. Trying to persistently rid oneself of painful sensations, unwanted emotions, distressing memories or unpleasant thoughts leads one away from their personally

chosen values—the activities that are desired and meaningful. This experiential avoidance contributes to **psychological inflexibility** and causes suffering.[13]

In many ways, ACT challenges conventional methods of pain management that focus on pain control and symptom reduction. At times, it may feel different than traditional cognitive behavioral therapy or the more recent pain education approaches. These cognitive behavioral therapies aim to change pain-related cognitions, challenge pain-related beliefs, restructure thoughts, provide education where it is lacking, and use motivational incentives to reduce fear, pain and other symptoms.[14] The suggestion is that when fear and pain-related thoughts are reduced, the patient no longer needs to avoid a situation and can behave more effectively. This approach has been acknowledged as one of the safest and most effective treatment approaches for chronic pain.[15]

Indeed, traditional cognitive behavioral therapy for chronic pain has been successful in many ways. Yet traditional cognitive behavioral approaches for pain report small benefits for disability, mood and catastrophic thinking in trials that compared cognitive behavioral therapy with no treatment, and long-term benefits often wane.[16] Similarly, modern pain education approaches purport to assist patients to reconceptualize their pain away from a biomedical cause and towards a more biopsychosocial understanding.[17] This approach aims to change or modify thoughts and beliefs about the cause of pain and has added to our cognitive methods of treating pain. However, varying degrees of reconceptualization exist with most patients showing only partial reconceptualization.[18] Our ability to change pain-related thoughts and beliefs is often patchy, and people are left suffering. Further methods to help people with both their inner experiences related to thoughts,

feelings and sensations as well as their outer world behavior is desirable.

ACT shows us that emotional responses such as fear, pain-related thoughts and memories from a person's unique learning history cannot be changed nor completely eliminated. There is no delete button in the nervous system to erase what's been learned. The strong possibility remains that some life event will occur in the future where these same feelings and thoughts yet again influence behavior. ACT does not attempt to change thoughts or beliefs and it is not pain relief focused. Although pain relief may occur, it is not an absolute prerequisite for vital living. Clinically, there is minimal interest in what is true or false about pain in any sense (e.g., when clients struggle to determine whether their thoughts or beliefs about their back pain is or is not caused by a herniated disc). Instead, there is a great interest in workability (e.g., how is it working for the individual to struggle to determine whether his or her thoughts or beliefs about back pain are correct?) It can be difficult to think or talk oneself out of a situation created by thinking and talking. Education, logic and instruction may have limits in cultivating the processes of behavior change.

Infusing ACT into Physical Therapy and Other Health Professions

ACT has been shown to have positive effects on chronic pain, and meta-analyses show improvements in depression, anxiety, pain intensity, pain interference, physical functioning and quality of life.[19, 20, 21] This has made it attractive for mental health and physical medicine professionals alike. A wide variety of health professionals can use ACT to inform their treatment of pain, and it cuts across specialties. This includes physical therapists, occupational therapists, nurses, physicians, health coaches, and of course, mental health professionals.

Physical therapy is often the first point of entry into the healthcare system for people experiencing pain. The non-invasive and non-pharmacologic approach taken by physical therapists towards the treatment of pain makes the profession ideally suited to adopt evidence-based therapies of psychologically-informed practice. Treatments based on principles of cognitive behavioral therapy, including acceptance and commitment therapy, delivered by professionals other than psychologists continue to flourish and show promise.[22, 23, 24] Within a self-management approach, physical therapists can weave principles of ACT into practice and effectively address the psychological distress associated with chronic pain.[25]

With sufficient training and ongoing mentorship, physical therapists and other health professionals can implement ACT alongside other types of therapies, including pain education and exercise therapy.[26] It can be used face-to-face, via telehealth, in individual or group programs. Professionals can choose from brief time-limited interventions for busy primary musculoskeletal practice or implement full protocols guided by the core processes. Across a wide range of conditions, practitioners and practice settings, ACT seeks a unified model of behavior change.[27]

How to Use This Book

My aim with this book is to provide you with a personal experience of the foundational exercises and techniques used to treat pain. Throughout the book, each chapter presents opportunities to learn, practice, and cultivate the processes that support psychological flexibility. It is strongly recommended you read the entire book from cover to cover and practice before you start using any of it with a patient.

As you read the book, set aside time each day to experience the exercises on your own. Each chapter includes one or two exercises, activities or questions to contemplate. A chapter each day is a good pace for which to work through the material. Other than what is discussed in this section the theory, technical terms and footnotes have been mindfully omitted. Not only does this free you from the complexity of theory, but most importantly, allows you to experience ACT as would a patient. There is also a lot of useful information about this science on the website for the Integrative Pain Science Institute, which is focused on the development of the work I write about in this book: **www.integrativepaininstitute.com.**

Engaging in this process can help you determine what areas to focus on next in terms of learning ACT and improving your skills. Therapists come to ACT from all different professions and with a variety of skill and knowledge. How best to learn ACT has not been well studied although experts agree that an intensive educational training with monthly supervision is ideal.[28]

REFERENCES

1. Bendelow G. (2013). Chronic pain patients and the biomedical model of pain. *The virtual mentor : VM*, 15(5), 455–459. https://doi.org/10.1001/virtualmentor.2013.15.5.msoc1-1305

2. Sullivan M. D. (2018). Depression Effects on Long-term Prescription Opioid Use, Abuse, and Addiction. *The Clinical journal of pain*, 34(9), 878–884. https://doi.org/10.1097/AJP.0000000000000603

3. Meints, S. M., & Edwards, R. R. (2018). Evaluating psychosocial contributions to chronic pain outcomes. *Progress in neuro-psychopharmacology & biological psychiatry*, 87(Pt B), 168–182. https://doi.org/10.1016/j.pnpbp.2018.01.017

4. Edwards, R. R., Dworkin, R. H., Sullivan, M. D., Turk, D. C., & Wasan, A. D. (2016). The Role of Psychosocial Processes in the Development and Maintenance of Chronic Pain. *The journal of pain : official journal of the American Pain Society*, 17(9 Suppl), T70–T92. https://doi.org/10.1016/j.jpain.2016.01.001

5. Hayes, S. C., Strosahl, K. D., & Wilson, K. G. (2012). *Acceptance and commitment therapy: The process and practice of mindful change* (2nd ed.). Guilford Press.

6. Vowles, K. E., Witkiewitz, K., Levell, J., Sowden, G., & Ashworth, J. (2017). Are reductions in pain intensity and pain-related distress necessary? An analysis of within-treatment change trajectories in relation to improved functioning following interdisciplinary acceptance and commitment therapy for adults with chronic pain. *Journal of consulting and clinical psychology*, 85(2), 87–98. https://doi.org/10.1037/ccp0000159

7. Hayes, S. C., Barnes-Holmes, D., & Roche, B. (Eds.). (2001). *Relational Frame Theory: A Post-Skinnerian account of human language and cognition*. New York: Plenum Press.

8. Wicksell, R. K., & Vowles, K. E. (2015). The role and function of acceptance and commitment therapy and behavioral flexibility in pain management. *Pain Management*, 5(5), 319-322. doi:10.2217/pmt.15.32

9. ayes, S. C., Hofmann, S. G., Stanton, C. E., Carpenter, J. K., Sanford, B. T., Curtiss, J. E., & Ciarrochi, J. (2019). The role of the individual in the coming era of process-based therapy. *Behaviour Research and Therapy*, 117, 40– 53. https://doi.org/10.1016/j.brat.2018.10.005

10. Feliu-Soler A, Montesinos F, Gutiérrez-Martínez O, Scott W, McCracken LM, Luciano JV. Current status of acceptance and commitment therapy for chronic pain: a narrative review. *J Pain Res*. 2018;11:2145-2159 https://doi.org/10.2147/JPR.S144631

11. McCracken, L. M., & Gutiérrez-Martínez, O. (2011). Processes of change in psychological flexibility in an interdisciplinary group-based treatment for chronic pain based on Acceptance and Commitment Therapy. *Behaviour Research and Therapy*, 49(4), 267-274. doi:https://doi.org/10.1016/j.brat.2011.02.004

12. A-Tjak, J. G. L., Davis, M. L., Morina, N., Powers, M. B., Smits, J. A. J., & Emmelkamp, P. M. G. (2015). A Meta-Analysis of the Efficacy of Acceptance and Commitment Therapy for Clinically Relevant Mental and Physical Health Problems. *Psychotherapy and Psychosomatics*, 84(1), 30-36. doi:10.1159/000365764

13. Gentili, C., Rickardsson, J., Zetterqvist, V., Simons, L. E., Lekander, M., & Wicksell, R. K. (2019). Psychological Flexibility as a Resilience Factor in Individuals With Chronic Pain. *Frontiers in psychology*, 10, 2016. https://doi.org/10.3389/fpsyg.2019.02016

14. Sturgeon J. A. (2014). Psychological therapies for the management of chronic pain. *Psychology research and behavior management*, 7, 115–124. https://doi.org/10.2147/PRBM.S44762

15. Ehde, D. M., Dillworth, T. M., & Turner, J. A. (2014). Cognitive-behavioral therapy for individuals with chronic pain: efficacy, innovations, and directions for research. *The American psychologist*, 69(2), 153–166. https://doi.org/10.1037/a0035747

16. Williams, A., Eccleston, C., & Morley, S. (2012). Psychological therapies for the management of chronic pain (excluding headache) in adults. *Cochrane Database of Systematic Reviews*(11). doi:10.1002/14651858.CD007407.pub3

17. Moseley, L. (2007). Reconceptualising pain according to modern pain science. *Physical Therapy Reviews*, 12, 169-178. doi:10.1179/108331907X223010

18. King, R., Robinson, V., Ryan, C. G., & Martin, D. J. (2016). An exploration of the extent and nature of reconceptualisation of pain following pain neurophysiology education: A qualitative study of experiences of people with chronic musculoskeletal pain. *Patient education and counseling*, 99(8), 1389–1393. https://doi.org/10.1016/j.pec.2016.03.008

19. Hughes, L. S., Clark, J., Colclough, J. A., Dale, E., & McMillan, D. (2017). Acceptance and Commitment Therapy (ACT) for Chronic Pain: A Systematic Review and Meta-Analyses. *The Clinical journal of pain*, 33(6), 552–568. https://doi.org/10.1097/AJP.0000000000000425

20. Veehof, M. M., Trompetter, H. R., Bohlmeijer, E. T., & Schreurs, K. M. (2016). Acceptance- and mindfulness-based interventions for the treatment of chronic pain: a meta-analytic review. *Cognitive behaviour therapy*, 45(1), 5–31. https://doi.org/10.1080/16506073.2015.1098724

21. Vowles, K. E., Pielech, M., Edwards, K. A., McEntee, M. L., & Bailey, R. W. (2019). A Comparative Meta-Analysis of Unidisciplinary Psychology and Interdisciplinary Treatment Outcomes Following Acceptance and Commitment Therapy for Adults with Chronic Pain. *The journal of pain : official journal of the American Pain Society*, S1526-5900(19)30841-7. Advance online publication. https://doi.org/10.1016/j.jpain.2019.10.004

22. Barker, K. L., Heelas, L., & Toye, F. (2016). Introducing Acceptance and Commitment Therapy to a physiotherapy-led pain rehabilitation programme: an Action Research study. *British Journal of Pain*, 10(1), 22–28. https://doi.org/10.1177/2049463715587117

23. Hall, A., Richmond, H., Copsey, B., Hansen, Z., Williamson, E., Jones, G., Fordham, B., Cooper, Z., & Lamb, S. (2018). Physiotherapist-delivered cognitive-behavioural interventions are effective for low back pain, but can they be replicated in clinical practice? *A systematic review. Disability and rehabilitation*, 40(1), 1–9. https://doi.org/10.1080/09638288.2016.1236155

24. Silva Guerrero AV, Maujean A, Campbell L, Sterling M. A Systematic Review and Meta-Analysis of the Effectiveness of Psychological Interventions Delivered by Physiotherapists on Pain, Disability and Psychological Outcomes in Musculoskeletal Pain Conditions. *Clin J Pain*. 2018;34(9):838-857. doi:10.1097/AJP.0000000000000601

25. Hutting, N., Johnston, V., Staal, J. B., & Heerkens, Y. F. (2019). Promoting the Use of Self-management Strategies for People With Persistent Musculoskeletal Disorders: The Role of Physical Therapists. *The Journal of orthopaedic and sports physical therapy*, 49(4), 212–215.

26. Casey, M. B., Smart, K., Segurado, R., Hearty, C., Gopal, H., Lowry, D., Flanagan, D., McCracken, L., & Doody, C. (2018). Exercise combined with Acceptance and Commitment Therapy (ExACT) compared to a supervised exercise programme for adults with chronic pain: study protocol for a randomised controlled trial. *Trials*, 19(1), 194. https://doi.org/10.1186/s13063-018-2543-5

27. Hayes S. C. (2019). Acceptance and commitment therapy: towards a unified model of behavior change. *World psychiatry: official journal of the World Psychiatric Association* (WPA), 18(2), 226–227. https://doi.org/10.1002/wps.20626

28. Walser, R. D., O'Connell, M., Coulter, C.(2019) *The Heart of ACT: Developing a Flexible, Process-Based, and Client-Centered Practice Using Acceptance and Commitment Therapy.* Context Press

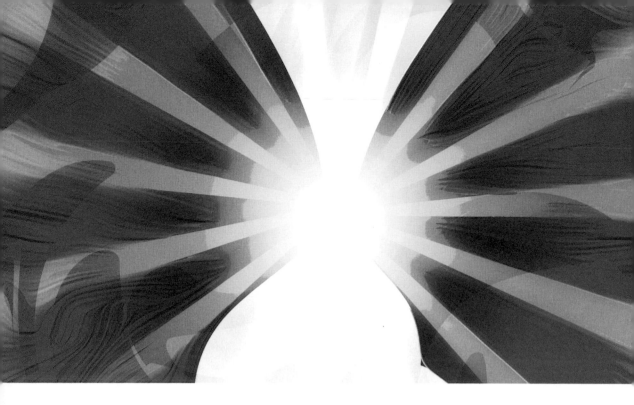

PART I

Learning About Pain:
The More We Understand, The Less We Suffer

"That danger message arrives at the brain and the brain has to decide:
What does this mean? What should be done here?"
– Lorimer Moseley

CHAPTER 1: UNDERSTANDING PAIN

This chapter is the beginning of your journey and requires you to put on your thinking cap. It may seem like a radical idea to suggest that learning about pain is one of the most effective ways to overcome it. But it's true; knowledge is powerful pain medicine, and it can help you return to a rich, full life. Long-term chronic pain interferes with the ability to enjoy almost everything life has to offer. From being productive at work, to spending quality time at home, or enjoying friends and hobbies—pain makes a great dent in the sense of joy, meaning and purpose that life offers. When pain intensifies or persists, it takes up space and may occupy every waking moment. Understanding pain and knowing *why* you hurt can help tremendously. Have you ever had any of the following thoughts related to pain? "Why am I in pain?" Why has this pain lasted so long?" "Pain gets in the way of everything!" "I could do _____

_____

_____

_____ if I didn't have this pain!"

Overcoming pain is possible, and getting your life back begins with learning how pain works. The latest research shows the more you understand about pain, the better your chance of overcoming it. The more information that is shared with people living with pain, the greater the chance of returning to a full and active life. It doesn't require special medical training and you don't need to be a whiz kid; anyone can do this. Knowledge about pain improves how people live, and facts ease fear, empowering people to take action and live better. This chapter will cover the most important facts about the new science of pain.

Many people view pain as a bother and spend an enormous amount of time searching for answers as to why they still hurt, and for good reason. Modern pain remedies make it seem as if we can just wave a magic wand and make all pain go away. Have you tried remedies that make such a claim? Have they worked? The truth is, pain serves an important function and is a necessary part of life. Without it, you wouldn't feel the prick of a sewing needle or a rock in your shoe. If you enjoyed a shower this morning and adjusted the hot and cold water to just the right temperature, your ability to feel pain was at work. It protected you from burning yourself. If you recently broke an ankle, pain told you not to walk or place weight on your foot. And going a little deeper, there is no love without the possibility of pain. Pain is a part of life.

Old pain treatments centered on repairing bones, muscles, joints and other tissues. If you have ever had a papercut or broken a bone, both are examples of an injury that required the tissues to heal. The human body knows how to solve this problem. When injured, it coordinates a rapid response and the immune system goes to work repairing any tissue that was damaged. You are already familiar with this process, having experienced some of life's common bruises, bumps and breaks. From a scraped knee while learning to walk, to a torn tendon from playing tennis, all damaged tissues in the body heal within six months. This is **pain fact #1: All tissues in the body heal within six months.** This is true no matter what the injury, no matter how severe it is, and no matter what the most recent pain doctor or guru has told you. It may be assumed that once you reach the six-month point, it's smooth sailing from there on out. The myth from the old pain model is that as tissues heal, the pain subsides, you start to move more easily, and you eventually return to the life you once enjoyed. This is only half the story.

If you are reading this book, there is a good chance the above scenario hasn't played out so neatly. You've probably struggled with pain that has lasted far more than six months. It may even be years or decades that pain has weighed you down like a heavy ball and chain. You may be thinking, "I've had pain much longer than six months; why do I still hurt?" The answer can be found in the new science of pain and by discovering the important distinction between acute pain (short-term) and chronic (long-term) pain.

Long-term, or chronic pain, lasting for more than six months, has less to do with the tissues (muscles, bones and joints). Nowhere is this more obvious than in the large number of people who suffer from chronic low back pain or fibromyalgia. Decades of imaging studies have revealed that X-rays and MRI findings rarely corroborate with one's report of pain. Many people have no observable findings of tissue injury on imaging studies but have severe unrelenting back pain. There are also people who report no pain but have images that show damage. This tells us chronic pain means much more than an injury that hasn't healed properly. In fact, over a third of people living with pain report no injury at all! How can that be? How can there be pain without an injury? **Pain fact #2** points us toward the discovery that: **Pain and tissue injury are two separate issues**. Pain can be its own condition, separate from any tissue damage. Even if you blew out your knee while playing college football or sustained whiplash in a car accident (only about 25% of people with whiplash go on to report long-term pain), pain alone is a poor indicator of tissue damage. This is **pain fact #3: Worse injuries don't always result in worse pain**.

We are only into the first chapter and already you know more about chronic pain than most practitioners. During our short time together, we've covered some of the most important facts that spark curiosity, alleviate some of the worries about reinjury, and can power you to keep moving forward. So far, we know:

- All tissues in the body heal within six months.
- Pain and tissue injury are two separate issues.
- Worse injuries don't always result in worse pain.

Like pain researchers, if we look at the new science of pain and collect the facts, they point us away from the tissues as the guilty culprit. There are still unanswered questions about what causes pain. How can pain possibly occur if the tissues are not the cause? This leads us to **pain fact #4: The brain generates pain, not the body's tissues**. Despite what you have been told, the brain—not the body—creates pain. Let's take a closer look at how this works.

It is a myth that there are pain signals or pain pathways in the body. An important distinction to make here is that the nervous system carries messages, not pain. The body's network of nerves is responsible for transmitting messages up to the brain. As the brain receives this information it decides if action is needed to prevent harm (like quickly removing your foot from that sharp tack on the floor). Some messages carry danger, other messages carry safety. Danger messages are a vital part of evolution that serve to protect us. The danger messages from the body's tissues send the message to the brain. The brain then determines, based on all credible evidence, whether the body needs protection. This system is essential to your survival and keeps you safe. Pain is about protection!

Once these messages arrive at the brain, the brain decides whether or not to create pain. Pain is produced based on the threat of danger or harm. The scientific name for these messages is nociception. Pain and *nociception* are different phenomena. Pain cannot be inferred solely from activity in neurons. But remember, you don't have to be a pain scientist to understand pain!

Sometimes messages are sufficient to produce pain. Sometimes messages do not produce pain, like when you bump your thigh on the coffee table and notice a black and blue bruise days later. What happened here? In this example, the black and blue bruise represents tissue damage but there is no pain! The brain wasn't concerned about a little bump that caused a bruise. Pain comes from the brain, and nerves carry messages from the body to the brain to alert it of danger.

If nerves continuously deliver danger messages over a long period of time, they keep sounding the *harm alarm*. Over time, the brain and nervous system may become sensitive and hyper-responsive to these danger messages. *This* causes the nervous system to become overly sensitive. An overly sensitive nervous system creates pain, even in times of absolutely no danger. It is constantly on guard and on high alert. How can you tell if the nervous system is overly sensitive? Here are some ways to measure. (Check off those that apply to you.)

☐ Pain is unpredictable.

☐ Mood changes occur due to pain.

☐ Pain flares even after mild activity.

☐ Pain has persisted beyond six months.

☐ Pain is linked to certain people, places, or events.

☐ Pain spreads, moves, or occurs in multiple body parts.

☐ Pain is linked to certain thoughts, emotions or feelings.

☐ Many different types of activity or movement trigger pain.

☐ Hobbies, housework or exercise are avoided due to pain.

☐ Pain is linked with a previous trauma (physical or emotional).

☐ Thoughts of physical activity or reinjury cause fear or anxiety.

What causes nerves to continually create danger messages is the million-dollar question and one scientists have been studying for decades. Pain is always a personal experience that is influenced to varying degrees by biological, psychological and social factors. Anything in your environment that signals harm has the potential to create pain. As the brain processes pain, your thoughts, emotions, beliefs and behavior play an extraordinary role. Thoughts and emotions can produce danger messages, especially with regard to how you feel about pain and how you relate to it. This leads us to **pain fact #5: Chronic pain is due to a sensitive nervous system and our thoughts, emotions and behavior play a role**. This is one of the reasons we begin with learning about pain. The best science shows that when people living with pain understand how the nervous system and brain produce pain they experience less discomfort, are less afraid, more physically active and do more of what they love.

We've learned a lot about pain in very little time. Let's take a moment and review the most important points.

Pain fact #1: All tissues in the body heal within six months.

Pain fact #2: Pain and tissue injury are two separate issues.

Pain fact #3: Worse injuries don't always result in worse pain.

Pain fact #4: The brain generates pain, not the body's tissues.

Pain fact #5: Chronic pain is due to a sensitive nervous system and our thoughts, emotions and behavior play a role.

🧠 Take the quiz to test your knowledge thus far:

1. **All tissues in the body heal within six months.**

☐ True   ☐ False

Answer: True. When an injury occurs, the immune system coordinates a rapid response and repairs all damaged tissues. This is true no matter what the injury or how severe. All tissues in the body heal within six months.

2. **An injury isn't necessary for pain to develop.**

☐ True   ☐ False

Answer: True. Old pain treatments centered on the repair of bones, muscles, joints and other tissues. The newest pain science has revealed that chronic pain is due to a sensitive nervous system and our thoughts, emotions and behavior play a role. It is possible to have pain without sustaining an injury.

3. **The body tells the brain when it is in pain.**

☐ True   ☐ False

Answer: False. The body's network of nerves is responsible for transmitting messages to the brain. As the brain receives these messages it decides whether or not to create pain. The body doesn't tell the brain when it is in pain. It is the brain's decision to produce pain.

4. **Chronic pain means an injury hasn't healed.**

☐ True   ☐ False

Answer: False. Long-term or chronic pain lasting for more than six months has little to do with the tissues. Many people have no observable findings of tissue damage on imaging studies but have severe unrelenting pain. Decades of imaging studies have revealed that X-rays and MRI findings rarely corroborate with one's report of pain. Chronic pain means much more than an injury that hasn't healed properly. Chronic pain is due to a sensitive nervous system and our thoughts, emotions and behavior play a role. Pain and nociception are different phenomena. Pain cannot be inferred solely from activity in sensory neurons.

5. **Worse injuries always result in worse pain.**

☐ True   ☐ False

Answer: False. Pain is a poor indicator of tissue damage. Worse injuries don't always result in worse pain. Some people have no injury and still have pain.

If you are enjoying learning about pain there is still more to learn. We can learn more from this definition of chronic pain, published by the great minds at the International Association for the Study of Pain. They define pain as, "an unpleasant sensory and emotional experience associated with, or resembling that associated with, actual or potential tissue damage." Whoa, that's a mouthful for any pain scientist to explain! Let's unpack this definition and break down each part of the sentence and see how it supports what we've learned so far:

"Pain is an unpleasant sensory and emotional experience"
Anyone who has suffered from pain can tell you that it hurts in your body (that's the sensory part) and there is an undeniable component that it impacts our thoughts and mood (that's the emotional part). This supports **pain fact #5: Chronic pain is due to a sensitive nervous system and our thoughts, emotions and behavior play a role**.

"associated with actual tissue damage"
Some of you reading this may have had an injury—which is actual tissue damage. Some of you may have had minor injuries that caused severe pain. Some of you, with what may seem like awful injuries, have very little pain. Even two of the exact same injuries can have different pain outcomes in different people. This part of the definition supports **pain fact #3: Worse injuries don't always result in worse pain**. Finally, we know from **pain fact #1: All tissues in the body heal within six months**.

"resembles potential tissue damage"
This part means that there is no distinction between the way pain operates in people who have a recent injury, those who have no injury, and those who had injuries that healed long ago. Injury or tissue damage is not needed for pain. **Pain fact #2: Pain and tissue injury are two separate issues** and **pain fact #4: The brain generates pain, not the body's tissues**.

It's important to clarify a few points:
Chronic pain no longer serves a protective role and it may have adverse effects on function, social and psychological wellbeing. But even though pain is caused by the brain, and is a subjective experience, something crucial is missing from the definition. Just because pain is produced by the brain doesn't mean you are making it up. **Your pain is 100% real**. A person's report of pain should be respected. Through personal life experiences, individuals learn the concept of pain.

Those who are up-to-date on the latest science understand you are not fabricating it. Because pain is invisible, people sometimes jump to the conclusion that people are fabricating pain. Still today, many of our highest credentialed practitioners subscribe to the outdated belief that if there is no observable injury then the person is making it up. Worse, pain is sometimes labeled as a mental health condition that must be treated with antidepressants and antianxiety medications. This has led to a stigma around pain. Pain is not a mental health condition. It's time to raise awareness around the proper treatment and how poorly our industrialized medical-pharmaceutical system treats pain, all while making billions of dollars, without truly helping many people.

Your pain is real and chronic pain can be treated by learning how pain works, how the mind works, and by making behavior changes that can help move you toward a more meaningful and purpose-filled life. This shift in thinking about pain helps patients and practitioners alike. A new idea is the spark that lights an eternal flame. The more you know, the easier it is to overcome pain. Take a moment to skim this chapter again. On the next page, write down three new or surprising details you learned about pain. People who understand how pain works live better. In the next chapter, we'll learn more about how pain works to protect us.

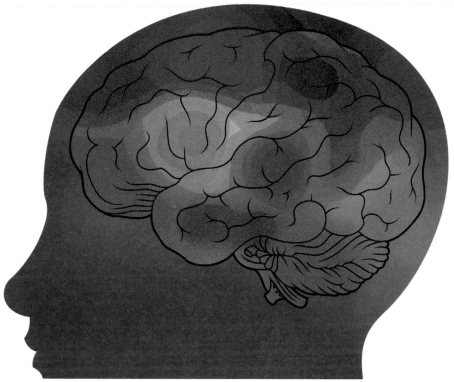

Pain research has shown that the brain generates pain, not the body's tissues.

What Did I Learn Today?

Write 1-3 things you learned today that can be used this week.

1._____
_____
_____

2._____
_____
_____

3._____
_____
_____

CHAPTER 2: THE PROTECTOR WITHIN

In the first chapter, we covered the basics about the new science of pain. Hopefully, this knowledge has begun to settle in, and you have had a few "a-ha" moments. You may even have already experienced a breakthrough on your journey. Learning that chronic pain is not just about the muscles, tendons and joints and that it's a condition of the nervous system can impact how you think about and experience pain. For some, this foundational information is enough to dispel the looming threat of pain, ease fear and worry, and sometimes even decrease pain. Once you understand that the pain you feel does not equal tissue damage, you're one step closer to being more active and living better.

Yet, through decades of treating patients experiencing pain, I've discovered that there's one thing that always seems to stand in the way of a patient's full recovery and return to an active life: The human mind and all its thinking. Logically, you may fully or partially understand the concept of a sensitive nervous system but still may not be able to stop thinking and worrying about pain and your physical body. If this is the case, the common impulse is to either control pain, to avoid pain at any cost, or to get hooked into thinking about pain—focusing on it through rumination and worry and allowing it to take charge of your inner life.

Even for those familiar with modern pain science, who understand that pain does not equal damage, the protective and problem-solving part of the mind may continue to warn of danger. Why is our human mind so attentive to pain? I call this aspect of our mind the **Protector Within** because it is constantly suggesting solutions to control physical and psychological pain, even though our own experience may suggest otherwise.

This voice within means no harm and is, in fact, concerned about your safety. Although, if you pay attention and listen to the solutions it urges you to seek, rarely are they suggestions that promote long-term health, and some are downright harmful. The Protector Within has a powerful impulse to problem-solve the pain away. When you see how the Protector does what it does, you are closer to finding relief—a radical form of relief—that will help in almost every area of your life.

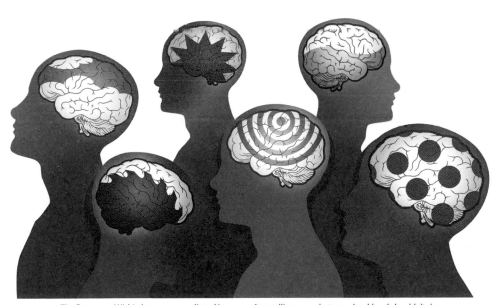

The Protector Within has a personality of its own, often telling you what you should and shouldn't do.

The Protector Within may be telling you a story about your pain and what is true or not true about your pain. It may remind you of other people's opinions and recommendations, even if they're outdated and you know they aren't healthy. And, if the Protector Within is not satisfied with a practitioner's opinion, it will encourage you to seek a second opinion from a new, more qualified expert. It can lure you to the couch for a midday catnap or encourage you to pour an extra drink in the evening as a proven way to soothe pain. If left unchecked, it has the potential to lead you down a dangerous path with grave consequences, including the misuse of opioids, which has become a global health crisis.

Controlling and avoiding pain seems logical to the Protector Within. Always working, it brings all potential problem-solving tools to the table. Unfortunately, this can lead to rigid problem-solving "solutions," such as, "get rid of it," "cut it out," "repair it," or, "rest."

During the Stone Age, listening to the voice within to avoid pain was a vital survival instinct. Responding to the message, "Get your hand out of the sabretooth tiger's mouth!" or following the mind's direction to "Fight!" or "Flee!" when an enemy tribe is on the attack, is important to survival. Ignoring these messages could cost your life. However, in the modern world—where we know pain is both a physical and psychological experience involving thoughts and emotions—it's completely different. The messages we tell ourselves, through the voice of the Protector, are not heard simply as things we're thinking but as hard truths.

Each of us has a Protector Within and it may take many forms, sounding different from day to day. This voice within may be that of a helicopter parent, hovering over you, watching your every move as it looks out for your safety. This voice within may be that of a serious physician, listing medical facts and providing reasons why you should or shouldn't exercise. Your Protector Within may sound like a sweet grandmother, making sure you are safe and sound. Or, the voice within may sound dictatorial, bullying or using scare tactics to get you to follow its advice. Sometimes your Protector Within may annoy you, sometimes scare you, and at times might make you feel utterly vulnerable and helpless.

Your mind can be like one, or many, of these personalities. Here, you can benefit from getting some perspective by simply asking yourself, "Who's talking right now?" If the Protector Within were a person standing behind you, would you really want to listen to this person's suggestions or demands? If this seems too abstract, let's do an exercise to make it more concrete.

Humanizing the Protector Within

Begin by thinking about a specific movement or activity that causes you pain. It doesn't have to be something that causes extreme pain, but something that causes enough pain that you would want to avoid or stop it. You can do this with your eyes open or closed. Take a few minutes and imagine you're about to perform this activity.

What thoughts does your mind broadcast when you think about performing this activity? These messages are coming from your Protector Within. Next, imagine your Protector with as much detail as possible. How would you describe your Protector's personality? Is it caring, compassionate and loving, or impatient, strict and demanding? Would you enjoy chatting with and getting to know this voice within, or does your intuition tell you something is off?

Now, let's paint a clearer picture. Is your Protector male or female? How tall is your Protector? What age is he or she? If your Protector had a face, what would it look like? What type of clothes are they wearing? What is the tone of your Protector's voice? Is it positive, soft and soothing? Or, is it loud, forceful and angry?

Finally, take some time to reflect on the above questions and give your Protector a name or character description. This could be: Overprotective Parent, or Anxious Annie, or Albert the Know-it-all. Funny ones work well but use the description that you think fits best.

If your Protector Within were a real person, would you listen to everything they had to say about pain? Would you trust them to know what is best for you? Would you allow them to dictate where you go, what you do and with whom? Probably not. Use the following lines to describe your Protector Within.

My Protector's name is _____
_____.

My Protector looks like _____
_____.

My Protector's personality traits are _____
_____.

One thought my protector often broadcasts about pain is_____
_____.

Last, thank your Protector Within for being there and trying to help protect you. Thank your mind when you notice it butting in with thoughts, worries or opinions about pain and show some appreciation. For example, "Thank you for trying to protect me today!" You can also say, "Well, there goes my mind again," or, "My Protector is worrying again." Recognize that your Protector is simply your normal functioning mind. Knowing this, choose the kind of relationship you want to have with your Protector and how much leverage it has on what you do. This is called humanizing the mind, and it provides us with a window into our pain and how we relate to it.

CHAPTER 3: THE ILLUSION OF CONTROL

In the first chapter, we covered the latest science about chronic pain and how threats in our environment prime the nervous system to become sensitive. You also learned the brain determines whether you need protecting—pain is about protection! You are probably wondering, "Why did my nervous system stay sensitive and what can I do about it?" To answer these questions, we look at how the human brain evolved, how the mind works and the important role pain plays.

Back in the Stone Age, life was dangerous. For a caveman or cavewoman to survive, their minds had to constantly be on the lookout for things that might hurt them. In fact, if a cave person's mind wasn't good at predicting pain or spotting danger, what happened? They could have been killed by a neighboring tribe or eaten by a hungry tiger. The default setting of the caveman mind was safety first and pain meant grave danger. The caveman mind created thoughts like: "Watch out! There might be a tiger in that cave—you could get eaten," or, "Watch out! That enemy tribe on the horizon is racing toward you with sharp arrows—you could get killed!" Back in the Stone Age, surviving an encounter with a tiger was important information that was stored by the mind. The mind would store memories of past events and remember how pain was avoided, providing better preparation for next time. The caveman's mind evolved to pay close attention to pain. The caveman's mind evolved to warn us to avoid pain. This evolution has helped us live longer and become the dominant species on the planet. In fact, our minds are constantly problem-solving better ways to avoid pain.

As the human mind evolved it inherited this *protection from pain* as a priority. Although today we are unlikely to face a hungry tiger or an invading tribe. In fact, physical harm is rarely a problem. Modern threats are less about what is happening in the outside world and more about what each of us is experiencing in our inner world. The unpleasant thoughts, emotions and physical sensations we experience are what we fight and struggle to control. Once pain begins, the Protector Within asks questions such as, "How did this happen?" "How can this be controlled or eliminated?" "How do I get away from this?" It goes over painful memories, dwelling on them and reliving them, even when there's nothing useful to learn or the lesson was learned long ago. The evolved mind worries, predicts the worst and is constantly on the lookout for anything that might hurt or cause pain. The human mind evolved to work in such a way that it naturally creates psychological suffering. So, when your mind starts broadcasting unhelpful thoughts, as all minds do, remember it's not defective or abnormal. It's simply doing the job it evolved to do—keeping you safe from pain.

This is also why the medical system, and our culture at large, is all but obsessed with "feeling good." Look no further than the television where commercial breaks bombard us with advertisements about pills and promises to eliminate physical pain and its equal partner, psychological suffering. We have been taught from a young age that pain is undesirable, unacceptable, and we are to work to control it at all costs. Think about all the treatments you've tried or been recommended for pain. How many can you jot down? A short list might include opioid painkillers, anti-inflammatories, acupuncture, muscle relaxers, antidepressants, psychotherapy, exercise therapy, electric muscle stimulation, hypnosis, special supplements, surgery or injections. The message is that pain is bad, and you shouldn't have it. Yet, half of all people on disability are unable to work due to pain and a third of the globe struggles with chronic pain. We have more treatments for pain than ever in the history of human evolution, yet we live in a world full of pain. Have treatments designed to control pain worked?

As pain science has progressed, a significant amount of research shows that persistent attempts to avoid or control pain actually make pain worse. This means that many treatments and recommendations provided by most medical experts are actually not helpful, and a counterintuitive approach may be necessary. The treatments and recommendations given are feeding pain, not controlling it. Imagine that your pain is a small tiger kitten that you find at your front door one day. You play with him for a while and notice he is mewing nonstop. Your mind says, "Feed him, he must be hungry!" So, you feed him some raw beef—after all, that's what tigers love to eat! You do this every day, and each day your cute pet tiger grows a little bigger. As the little tiger's appetite grows, his daily meals change from hamburger meat to steak, to entire sides of beef. Your little pet no longer mews when hungry. Instead, he growls ferociously! He has turned into an uncontrollable, savage beast that will tear you apart if he doesn't get what he wants.

Our struggle with controlling, avoiding or trying to eliminate pain is similar. Every time you feed pain by attempting to control it, you help the pain-tiger grow larger and stronger. Controlling pain certainly seems like the sensible thing to do. It's what everyone has told you to do, and it makes sense from an evolutionary perspective. However, as you attempt to control pain, the pain-tiger growls ferociously—it wants more food. Yet, every time you feed it, the pain becomes stronger, more intimidating, and more controlling of your life. The problem with chronic pain is the danger message never stops. Over time, pain conditions you to think that something is wrong, and you need to control it. Pain is amplified by the fact that persistent attempts to control or avoid it causes more suffering.

The desire to control pain is built into the human nervous system, and our culture reinforces it. Avoidance in and of itself is not entirely bad; we all avoid pain to some extent. However, this becomes a problem when the avoidance strategies we've adopted get in the way of living a full life. When you adopt these avoidance strategies long term many of them interfere with living life to the fullest. Revisit the list of pain control or avoidance techniques you've tried—how many of them have worked to control pain long term? If you are like most people living with pain, probably not too many. More importantly, have any of these pain avoidance strategies kept you from living life to the fullest? Have your efforts to control or avoid pain caused your life to shrink down in some way? Have your efforts to control pain affected the life you dream of living? Sometimes our attempts to control pain cause additional pain and suffering. Our avoidance strategies can keep us from enjoying life by keeping us stuck in a struggle to avoid or control pain.

The Trouble With Pain Control

It would be great if we could simply flip the switch on pain to the permanent "off" position. From a young age, our culture tells us that we should be able to control many of our unpleasant and unwanted experiences. The idea that we are in control sounds appealing and works reasonably well when it comes to certain things we do—like deciding when to take a shower, pay the bills, or take the dog for a walk. The ability to control our outer world is what helped our cavemen ancestors from being eaten by lions, tigers and bears. If something threatening happens, we can take action. What's challenging is that control doesn't work so well when applied to the human mind, and our inner world of thoughts, emotions, memories or bodily sensations.

Think about the kinds of things we say to ourselves and each other when we are suffering and in pain. If it's physical pain: "Walk it off," "You can take it," "Put it out of your mind," or "Suck it up." For emotional pain and distress, such as worry, anxiety, sadness, fear and anger: "Don't worry about it," "Put it out of your mind," "Snap out of it," "Just don't think about it," or "Forget about it." Statements like these suggest that we have complete control of our inner experiences and that it is possible to dial down pain, switch off emotions or stop thoughts from occurring. Does the control each of us has over the outer world apply to our inner world? The following exercise will help you figure out the answer.

 Flip the Switch

Begin by sitting in a chair and focus all your attention on the following exercise:

- Pick any memory from yesterday and try to delete it. Go ahead. Press the delete button in your mind so you no longer have this memory.
- Next, make yourself as happy as possible. Try to flip on the happiness switch by really focusing on feeling happy. Don't cheat by thinking about a happy memory or looking at a photo from a happy event. Simply will yourself to feel happy.
- Now, get really mad without thinking of something that is frustrating or enraging.
- Focusing on your right thumb, make it go completely numb so that it can no longer move.
- Try really hard not to fill in the missing words. One, two, _____. Tic, tac,_____.
- Stop your mind from solving this problem. 1+1=_____.
- Without covering your eyes or ears, stop seeing or hearing.
- Finally, try and stop feeling pain wherever it may be.

How did you do? Were you able to successfully complete any tasks from the list above? These exercises help illustrate that many of our thoughts, emotions, memories and bodily sensations have no "off" switch. The human mind has no delete or erase button and evolved to be a problem-solving machine. To your mind, a problem is something that requires a solution. Pain becomes a problem to be solved, controlled or fixed.

Our problem-solving skills work so well in the outer world—like fixing a leaky pipe or a flat tire. It is only natural that the mind attempts to do the same with our inner world of thoughts, feelings, memories and bodily sensations. Unfortunately, when we try to control our inner experiences, it generally doesn't work. If it does work, it often gets in the way of living a full life, causing additional pain and suffering. Has trying to control thoughts, feelings, memories or bodily sensations made your pain better or worse? If you spend time, money and energy trying to control these inner sensations that are seemingly out of your control does it move you closer to the life you truly want? When you try to flip the "off" switch, you wind up thinking about pain even more, and it sensitizes the nervous system. Plus, it keeps you caught up in the fight to control pain instead of allowing you the freedom to enjoy life.

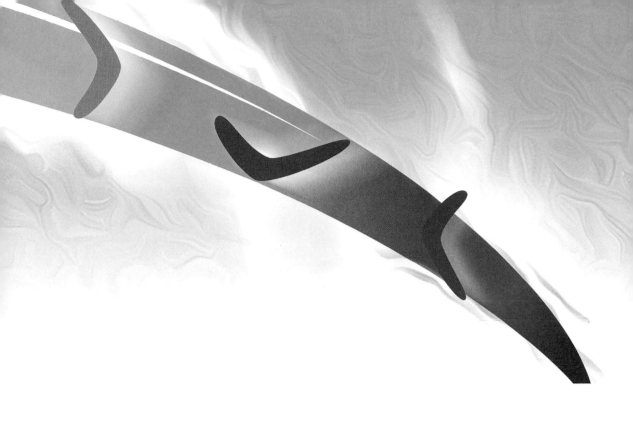

PART II

Stuck, Not Broken:
The Pivot to Being Open, Aware and Active

"Change the way you look at things and the things you look at change."
– Wayne Dyer

CHAPTER 4: FACING FEAR

Fear and pain can be useful in preventing acute injury by prompting you to take swift action to prevent trauma. Fear, like pain, is an essential emotion that serves to protect and keep you alive. Put simply, fear and pain are designed for survival. They keep you safe.

Fear and worry about pain roll in and break in waves. You may experience feelings of anxiety or impending danger. Thoughts about pain and the fear of damaging yourself further may flood your mind, and intense bodily sensations may rise such as tension in your shoulders, tightness in your chest, heart palpitations and shallow breathing. It may even feel like you are in the eye of a violent storm and on the verge of a panic attack.

Images and detailed pictures of painful events may also loop and replay like an old movie. These memories bubble up to the surface at the most inconvenient times, often when you are trying to move on with your life. You may find yourself caught in a cycle of avoiding pain, resting, obsessing over when it will return, and trying to distract or take your mind off the unpleasant feelings and emotions that come along for the ride. The proposition follows that pain is "all in your head" and can only be improved by changing how you think or changing what you believe about pain.

Fear about pain is normal, not a disorder. It is hardwired into human evolution. Mental health professionals have explored pain as a psychiatric disorder and have even tried to label pain as being a version of anxiety or depression. But pain is not a disease, or a psychiatric condition and you are not broken. What matters most is how you respond. Take a moment to consider: Is fear of pain a major problem in your life? If you answered yes, know you are not alone, and your response is normal.

Most people believe pain is the primary problem. They point to the location of the pain, rate the intensity of the pain, and describe how overwhelming and unrelenting it can be. Pain is unpleasant. But what if you take a step back and ask yourself: Is pain really the heart of the problem? Let's look closer at what makes pain a problem.

 ## What's the Problem?

Find a quiet place where you feel safe and won't be disturbed for a few minutes. Take some time to consider the following questions. Answer each question as openly and as whole-heartedly as possible. You can write your answers below. Pay attention to your fear of pain and ask yourself:

- How does my fear of pain interfere with my life?
- What activities do I avoid because I fear pain?
- What are the most troublesome aspects of my fear of pain?
- How does fear of pain keep me from living my best life?
- How does my fear of pain stand between me and the important things in my life?

> The thoughts, feelings, memories and sensations you most fear, the ones that make you want to hide, are the ones that need your attention and compassion. Facing and confronting pain-related fear by answering these questions is a great first step. Taking a step back and considering how fear restricts your life will help move you closer to who and what is most important to you.

CHAPTER 5: MINING FOR SOLUTIONS

Somewhere inside, a part of you knows that your best efforts to control pain haven't worked. It's likely that the struggle to control pain has cost you. Maybe you've experienced increased stress, missed time at work, canceled parties and opted out of social gatherings. It may be placing a strain on relationships with those you cherish most and could be leading you to "solutions" that cause negative effects on your health. Have you lost your freedom? Does pain feel like a barrier that's keeping you stuck?

Here's a metaphor that might describe how your situation feels: Imagine that you're standing in the middle of a large field and you're given a tool bag to carry. Your job is to walk out of the field and get home safely. Unbeknownst to you, the field contains a number of fairly deep holes that are hidden from sight. As you start walking toward home, eventually you fall into a deep hole. As hard as you try, you can't climb out. You search through the tool bag you were given; maybe it contains something you can use to get out of the hole. Now, suppose the only tool in the bag is a shovel. With no other options, you start trying to dig your way out. You're getting nowhere, but you're feeling frantic. So, you start digging faster. But you're still in the hole.

You're panicking. So, you try big shovelfuls, or little ones, or throwing the dirt far away, or not. Still, you are in the hole. All this effort and all this work, and oddly enough the hole has just gotten bigger and bigger and bigger. Does this sound similar to your experience with pain? Then you come to see me (or another health care professional) because you're thinking, "Maybe he has a huge shovel, a powerful steam shovel." Well, I don't. And even if I did I wouldn't use it, because digging is not a way out of the hole—it only makes the hole deeper. Are you digging right now?

People who are in pain can spend decades mining for solutions. They may start digging in one spot hoping for a solution, and then another spot, and then another, to no avail. The field of life becomes littered with holes. It's like a busy family of gophers creating a tunnel system hoping to hide and be protected from pain. Not only is the constant mining for a solution a problem but now your life is full of holes that you keep falling into.

The next exercise will help make you aware of the price you pay each time you search for a new solution. Notice the impact that your struggle to control pain has on each of these areas of your life. What have you opted out of, canceled, placed on hold or been unable to do because you were looking for solutions to control pain? In the activity below, write down a few examples in each area of your life, along with the cost it has had.

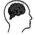 **Exploring the Costs**

What has pain cost financially? How much money have you spent on treatments in hopes of eliminating pain? Think of all the money you have spent on doctors' visits, medications, special supplements, massages and acupuncture. Consider the money you've spent on psychotherapy, exercise therapy, spiritual therapy, or other specialist treatment, self-help books and programs. What has the price been in terms of lost wages or missed days at work? Have you spent hundreds or thousands of dollars on expensive blood tests or imaging studies or on a quest for the next health guru or doctor to cure your pain?

What has pain cost emotionally? How much mental energy have you depleted worrying about pain, trying to solve pain or planning your life around pain in hopes of avoiding it? Does the accompanying anxiety or depression leave you feeling wired or tired, drained, frustrated or worn out? How has the struggle for pain control drained the battery of your energy reserves?

_____

What has pain cost your health? How have attempts to control pain affected your health? Do you have pain-related anxiety? Do you have the feeling of a constant knot in your stomach or irritable bowel syndrome? Do you have trouble concentrating, brain fog, problems falling asleep or staying asleep? Do you avoid exercise or normal daily activities because it might cause a pain flare-up? Do you indulge in sugary treats to self-soothe, possibly gaining excess weight that has made pain and movement more difficult? How has the medicine prescribed for your pain impacted your memory, concentration, focus, thinking, gut health or immune health?

_____

What has pain cost in your career? How has pain affected your work or career? Do you frequently come in late, leave early or call in sick due to pain? Has the quality of your work suffered, or have your coworkers commented on your lack of focus? Have you been passed over for a promotion? Has your boss noticed you have been preoccupied or less reliable lately? Have you quit a job or taken an extended medical leave due to pain?

_____

What has it cost in love and relationships? How has the struggle for pain control affected your social bonds? Have relationships with friends or family been strained or broken? Have you canceled or missed important family events or your children's important milestones such as birthdays or graduation? Has romance and intimacy with your partner or spouse been less frequent or absent? Are you unable to be a supportive parent, partner, friend or spouse? Have you isolated yourself or walled off from those you love?

_____

If the actions you've been taking to control pain are working, with no unwanted costs or negative consequences on your quality of life, then there is no problem. But if you are experiencing negative consequences, it's important to face the costs of pain on your life. It's important to feel the impact your struggle for pain control has had; this takes the bravery of a lion. Taking stock and reflecting on the five questions above can help create the momentum to move in a new life direction.

Completing this exercise often gives people an awareness of the amount of time, money, and energy they have spent on the quest for pain relief. They see, often for the first time, how the struggle for pain control is futile, and how it has made their life smaller. It provides an awareness of how the struggle for pain control can damage health, relationships and quality of life.

If you have a new awareness of the deep cost of pain, you are not alone and there is hope. You have arrived at a welcome sign at a fork in the road. This road has been crossed by many people on a journey to overcoming pain. Although you can't go back and change the past, you can move forward and create a new future from this very moment. You can learn to live beyond pain.

CHAPTER 6: THE PAIN TRAP

You likely purchased this book in hopes of finding a cure for your pain. This makes sense, as all the conventional messages about chronic pain recommend a reasonable amount of pain relief first, before you are able to return to life. This approach puts the cart before the horse and causes many to suffer unnecessarily. This book provides a fresh perspective and an alternate possibility that is backed by the latest science. If you continue to see pain as the primary problem, you just might miss the next train back toward a full and active life.

Sound radical? You don't have to trust me or the pain scientists. Look back at the list of the costs of trying to control or eliminate pain from the previous chapter. What has cost you more—living with pain or the countless pills, potions and promises to control or eliminate pain?

 Is Pain Control Working?

Take out a pen and paper for this exercise, or use the spaces provided below. Think about every treatment you've ever tried, or has been recommended to control or eliminate pain. Then, as openly and honestly as possible, answer the following questions.

Have the pain-management strategies worked to eliminate my pain? Think long term.

_____
_____.

Has the quest for pain control moved me closer to leading a more active life?

_____
_____.

Have the treatments cost me time, money, relationships, energy or caused even more pain?

_____
_____.

Have the treatments gotten in the way of the things I want to do or the people I deeply care about?

_____
_____.

Have the treatments helped me re-engage with the people and activities I find meaningful?

_____
_____.

It is like you are on a journey and when you arrive at the train station, two trains are waiting. One train is old and strange-looking, the seats are worn-out, and the inside looks dark, dingy and scary. On the next platform, there is a different train; it's a brand-new, shiny train; the latest in high-speed travel. It looks safe, reliable, the sort of train an executive traveling in first class might prefer. The sign says it has air conditioning, more legroom, free Wi-Fi, and a fancy lounge car with a free all-you-can-eat buffet. You think, "Wow! I just have to take this train, I couldn't possibly make my journey on that other jalopy, no way! This super train looks safe and comfortable." So, you wait for this "super" train to get ready to board and the old looking train goes on its way. You wait longer for the safe train and another old train leaves the station, and another, and yet another. All the while you are waiting for a chance to board this great, reliable train so you can take your journey, as yet another old looking one leaves. But here is the thing. What if the safe train can't ever board? What if it never leaves the station? What if you are waiting for the wrong train?

Years of research and clinical observation teach us that the struggle for pain relief is a trap. You've been trying to win the fight with pain, with fear of movement, with pain-related anxiety, true? Well, this approach is about letting the war roll on while you leave the battlefield. You've done exactly what anyone in your position would have done or tried. But the question you must ask yourself is, "Has the struggle to control pain worked, or has it created more problems?" Freedom from pain is found in letting go of the struggle for relief, because it may be causing more harm than good. It sucks up your time, money, resources, and places obstacles between you and the life you yearn to live. You're beginning to see a clearing through the forest, but only you can stop trying to control or eliminate pain. Choosing into this vulnerability helps free you from the pain trap.

CHAPTER 7: ENERGY HEALING

Things that are broken require fixing. When you view pain as a problem, it will naturally require a solution that promises to fix it. But what if the ways you've tried to mend or fix your pain are actually making things worse? Consider that possibility for a moment. Struggling to control pain can place a tremendous amount of strain on your body and your life. Each failed fix or promise of a solution to stop, control, or eliminate pain takes a toll. It lets you down, shattering your expectations into a thousand pieces, leaving you spent and drained of energy. In previous chapters, you've learned that your attempts to control or eliminate pain haven't fixed anything. The following metaphor will help you notice how ineffective the struggle with pain control really is. It also shows you a surprising alternate path out of the struggle—a path that can help you return to an active life.

 Letting Go of the Rope

The situation you are in is like being in a tug-of-war with a huge pain monster. In between you and this big, ugly monster is a deep, bottomless pit. Losing this tug-of-war means falling into the pit, where you'll be trapped forever. You grasp the rope tightly with both hands and begin to pull. The harder you pull, the harder the pain monster pulls back. You tighten your grip further until your knuckles are white. Your elbows contract and your shoulders rise with tension. Your back braces as you dig your heels into the ground and begin to pull. As the struggle continues you become more and more exhausted and begin to feel the pain in your body. Your arms are tired, your face is red and you're sweating as you continue in this fight for your life. As the struggle continues, you edge closer and closer to the pit. The pain monster is winning. Finally, you are pulled to the very edge of the pit where you stare into the depths of darkness. Your mind searches for solutions—telling you to pull harder and not to give in until you've won the struggle. Yet, there is an option you haven't considered; You don't need to win this tug of war. What if you decide to let go of the rope and give up the fight? Imagine yourself dropping the rope right now.

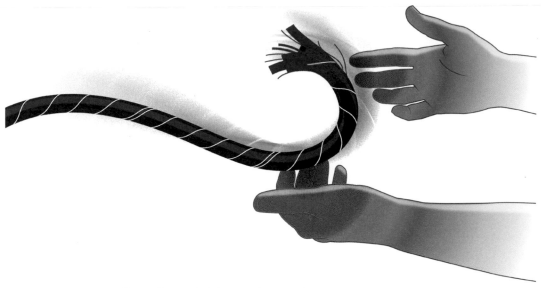

You can choose to drop the rope and free yourself from the struggle with pain.

Notice how your body feels as you drop the rope. Does the tension in your body increase or decrease? Does your energy level go up or down? You're now free to use your hands, feet, your entire body, and your mind for something other than fighting pain. The pain monster hasn't gone away just because you stopped tugging. He may still be holding one end hoping that you grab hold for another round. There may be times when you re-engage in this battle simply out of habit, even without the pain monster taunting you. By the time you complete this book, you will be better at noticing when you've grabbed the rope, allowing you to make the choice to let it go.

Dropping the rope will allow you to save your energy to focus on the important things you care about—relationships and activities that are waiting to be discovered or rediscovered. Goals and dreams that you have put on hold because you were busy in the battle with the pain monster. Take a moment and think about all the people and activities that have been waiting while you've been involved in the tug-of-war. What projects have you put on hold? What vacations have you canceled or put off planning? Is there a friend you no longer see or a child who needs your support? Start a list or simply visualize the people and places that make you feel excited about life again. How would dropping the rope give you more time, energy, and space to connect with who and what is important to you?

The difficult thing to realize is that your job is not to win the tug-of-war. Your job is to drop the rope. Letting go creates space for something new to take its place, or for something you once cherished to return. When you shift your focus from trying to control pain, worrying about when pain will return, or whether or not activities will cause more pain, you create space and energy to move toward the full and active life you desire. You are free to create the life you want.

CHAPTER 8: THE BOOMERANG EFFECT

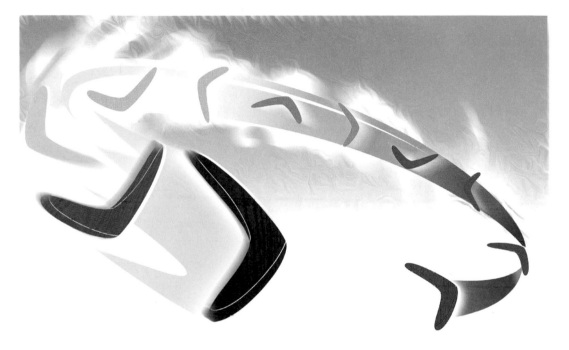

The more you push pain away, the harder it comes back—like a boomerang.

A boomerang is a curved throwing stick used by the aboriginal tribes of Australia for hunting and sport. Because of its unique aerodynamics, the boomerang returns to the thrower each and every time without fail. The more forceful you throw a boomerang, the faster and harder it comes back.

Responses to pain are often controlled by the yearning for relief, which can become a driving force in life. If controlling and avoiding pain become your overriding goal in life, you may find yourself in what I call the boomerang effect. Pain can increase the more you try to push it away. The greater the desire for pain relief, the greater the suffering, and the greater the intensity in return. In other words, the more you push pain away, the harder it comes back. That is the boomerang effect.

Pushing Pain Away

You can use your body as a way to experience the boomerang effect and to evaluate the impact it is having on your life. The strategies we use to control pain, or other unpleasant thoughts or emotions, can leave us feeling stuck and can pull us away from the people and activities that matter. They can also cause us to suffer. Let's explore this in a different way using the body.

Stand or sit very close to a solid, stable wall. Place your hands firmly against the wall at shoulder height (if you have a shoulder injury on one side use the other hand). Imagine that the wall represents all of the physical and emotional pain you want to control or eliminate from your life. Now begin to push gently against the wall, noticing that it doesn't budge. What are you feeling in your arms and shoulders? Next, push progressively harder against the wall, imagining you are pushing the pain away. As you continue to do this, notice any physical sensations in your arms, legs and torso. If you continued with this exercise for a prolonged period you would start to feel strained and fatigued. In addition to depleting your energy, think about how your life would be affected if you were pushing all day. How would you engage in activities that matter to you?

Continue pushing against the wall and consider how well you could complete things you need and want to do like nurturing your health, preparing a meal, helping a friend, volunteering at church, or contributing at work. When you are ready, stop pushing against the wall and notice the release of tension. How do your arms and body feel now?

You are the expert when it comes to your pain. Think about how you felt while pushing against the wall during this exercise. What did this experience teach you?

At times, we work hard trying to control pain and the unpleasant thoughts and emotions that accompany it. As hard as we might try to push away thoughts and emotions, it's impossible. It's like trying to hold an enormous inflatable beach ball under the water, but it keeps popping up out of the water. It's okay to allow the ball to float—simply let it be. Rather than stopping thoughts, we can stop fighting them. We can let thoughts be without reacting to them. When you're exhausting your energy trying to control or eliminate pain and it's not working, then it's time to try a radically different approach.

CHAPTER 9: GETTING UNSTUCK

As you travel on your journey to overcoming pain, you may find that your mind reverts to its old ways. The automatic pilot may turn on when you least expect it and old, unhelpful behaviors may unconsciously take control of your life. How can you turn off the autopilot of your mind? When you stop noticing, you can get stuck in patterns of reacting, shutting down and struggling.

If you were to get stuck in quicksand, your immediate impulse would be to struggle and fight to get out. But that's not what you should do in quicksand because as you put weight down on your feet, they sink deeper. The more you struggle, the deeper you sink, and the more you struggle. This is a no-win situation. Quicksand offers only one option for survival—lay out flat with your bodyweight spread over a large surface area. Although lying down and being with the quicksand goes against human instincts, it's exactly what is necessary for survival.

So it is with pain. As we struggle and fight against it, we may never have considered just letting go and being with the unpleasant thoughts, feelings, memories and sensations. If we did, we'd find we could get through it and survive more effectively than if we fought and struggled. Struggling against pain is like struggling in quicksand: The only way to survive is to stop struggling, spread out, and come into full contact with it.

 Let Yourself Go

Find a comfortable, seated position with your feet flat on the floor and your hands on your thighs. Close your eyes and bring awareness to your breath, noticing the rise and fall of each Inhalation and exhalation. Breathe in and out. Allow yourself to fully drop into this moment. Allow your shoulders, arms and legs to relax. Feel free to open your eyes at any time if you want.

Now, turn your attention to your pain, noticing any words or images that are associated with it. Continue breathing, thinking about one unpleasant word or one unpleasant image that you connect to your pain. Now, notice if you can observe these words and images while recognizing that you are separate from them. Take a long, deep breath in and out, allowing these thoughts and images to simply be what they are. If a word or image comes racing back, simply notice it, know you are not the word or image, take a deep breath and allow it to pass. If a word returns, name it, let it be and continuing breathing. Be aware that you now have this skill that you can use anytime life becomes difficult.

CHAPTER 10: YOUR INNER GPS

When you purchase a new car, it comes with detailed instructions on how to use its features, bells and whistles. It even provides safety tips and information about how to care for your vehicle to maintain its value. Most new cars come equipped with a state-of-the-art GPS for navigation. GPS, which stands for Global Positioning System, is a navigation system that tells you your exact location, 24 hours a day, in all weather conditions, anywhere in the world. A GPS makes navigation easier, allowing you to see where you are going, and preventing you from getting lost while keeping you on course. Unfortunately, life doesn't come with an owner's manual on how to navigate through persistent pain.

You likely picked up this book because you want help getting your life back on track after persistent, unrelenting pain has prevented you from living the life you want. Like an invasive vine, pain can grow into the cracks and permeate every aspect of your life. It can back you into a corner and make you feel like there is no way out. Consider all the ways pain has affected your life. Do you have to rest a lot and take frequent breaks? Are you missing out on quality time with people you care about? How has your overall health been impacted? Do everyday activities leave you feeling exhausted?

Many people with pain express a sense of loss. Some even say they *feel* lost. If your time and energy were once focused on friends, family, work, nurturing your health and participating in hobbies, but the day-in and day-out struggle to control or eliminate pain took over, it can feel like pain has taken the wheel and steered your life off course. It's like driving in a fog; you can't see the road ahead. Over time, it can affect your quality of life and make you feel as if life is fading away.

You've probably followed the advice of all the experts and taken the necessary steps to "manage" pain. Maybe you were told that when you learn to manage pain effectively, it will go down, and then you can start living. Yet, all you have is pain squeezing the life out of you. If controlling or eliminating pain isn't the answer, then what is? More importantly, what would a life free from pain look like?

You're at a fork in the road. The path leading to the right represents the road well-traveled. This smooth, well-paved road has been taken many times before. It's free of traffic, potholes, speed bumps and any other obstacles. It offers a safe route and you know where it leads—the coordinates are already programmed into your GPS. The signs on this road say it leads to complete pain relief, yet you never seem to get there.

The path to the left represents the road less traveled. This dirt road is filled with big, muddy potholes and is overgrown with grass and shrubs. You've avoided taking this unfamiliar road because it looks difficult to navigate, uncomfortable and scary—some parts may even appear a little treacherous. Now, what if I told you that everything that's important to you, everything and everyone you care deeply about in life lies along the bumpy road less traveled? Would you be willing to take this direction? What would make it worth exploring this route that you've never traveled before?

Now you have a choice. Which road will you take? Are you willing to take a difficult path, one that might involve some discomfort, if it means moving toward all that's meaningful to you? Instead of listening to your mind, I'm asking you to listen to your heart.

The first mile marker on the journey to overcoming pain is reconnecting with who and what you really care about. These are your values. In Acceptance and Commitment Therapy, we use the term "values" to refer to activities that give our lives meaning. Values are different than goals, in that we never "accomplish" a value. Instead, values are like a compass—they help us make choices based on the directions in which we want our lives to go.

Your unique and personally held values will guide you like the north star on your journey. Values keep you moving toward who and what is important, even when faced with difficult or unpleasant thoughts, emotions or sensations. Values are your inner GPS. They safely guide you day and night, rain or shine, through even the most turbulent storms. Values are less about the destination you seek, and more about the direction you are traveling.

Values include the personal qualities you choose to embody and help you be the person you want to be. They guide how you treat yourself and others and how you interact with the world around you. Values guide your actions and help you stay focused on what's important, helping you navigate on days when you feel pain, and on days when you feel great. They help you live the kind of life you want to live and be the kind of person you want to be.

Values are a highly evolved technology to navigate pain. It's time to plot a course and get back on track. There is a whole world to explore and rediscover—your friends, family, work, hobbies and community await. It's time to discover your values so you can start living by them. This exercise includes 10 questions to help you reconnect with who and what is most important to you. Chances are you have not thought about this because pain has occupied so much of your time and energy. Spend a few minutes thinking about each question before filling in the blank.

Valued Life Questions

What really matters to you, deep in your heart?

_____
_____

What sort of person do you want to be?

_____
_____

What personal strengths or qualities do you want to develop?

_____
_____

What does pain tell you about who really matters?

_____

_____

What important areas of life have you missed out on?

_____

_____

What does pain tell you about what really matters?

_____

_____

What in your life right now gives you a sense of meaning and purpose?

_____

_____

How can pain help you develop new skills?

_____

_____

How can pain help you grow as a person?

_____

_____

What matters to you in the "big picture" of life?

_____

_____

Which activities or people do you miss?

_____

_____

Freedom and overcoming pain involves recalibrating your GPS and taking one step in the direction toward who and what matters most, and then another. Which direction are you heading? You already have some knowledge and tools to guide you. What small action can you take today to move you closer?

PART III

Open Up and Observe:
Embrace All Experiences and See Thoughts
as They Are

"I used to think that the brain was the most wonderful organ in my body.
Then I realized who was telling me this."
— Emo Phillips

CHAPTER 11: NOTICING THOUGHTS

The idea of a Protector Within, introduced in Chapter 2, is a new concept. Humanizing the mind in this fashion is one way to begin to understand how the mind works and its influence on the way we live with pain. Because the Protector Within is concerned with safety, it tends to evaluate everything about ourselves and the events that occur in our lives, storing the information in our minds for later use. Why does the mind do this? When the mind stores details about events, it can make use of that information later on. This skill allows us to think about events, and experience them, even if we are not directly involved with them in the present moment. As a way to experience this at work, try the next exercise once you have read through the instructions.

Close your eyes and think of a big, juicy yellow lemon. Visualize a lemon as best as you can. Notice the bright yellow color, its shape, and the slightly bumpy texture of its skin. Next, imagine placing the lemon on a cutting board and with a knife slowly cutting into the skin and through the lemon until you have two halves. Now, imagine grabbing one half of the lemon with your hands and bring it up to your nose and smell it. Finally, imagine taking a bite into one half of the lemon and imagine its sweet but sour taste and the juice on the tip of your tongue.

What did you notice happen during that exercise as you imagined yourself biting into a bright yellow lemon? Chances are that you had a vivid image of a lemon, you could smell the lemon, you could taste it, and your mouth was probably bursting with saliva. If you dislike lemons you may have had a yucky feeling develop. This exercise shows us that even without actually having a lemon physically present, simply thinking about it is enough to have the same experience as if it were present. With this example in mind, consider what might happen if you replace the lemon with:

- Thoughts about pain
- Thoughts about movement and activity
- Thoughts about getting hurt
- Harsh judgments about yourself
- Memories of a past injury or a traumatic event
- Stories about the past or about pain

This little exercise shows that we can often react to an idea, image, or memory as if it were happening in the present moment. This ability to react to previously stored information has tremendous benefits and enables us to problem-solve. However, this human gift can also lead to problems. The trouble occurs when we automatically respond to our thoughts as if they were real. For example, the sudden thought "I have a weak right knee," can become confused with reality, and then we start to respond as though this is a fact. There is often a distinction between what our minds tell us and reality.

This may not seem like a problem, but the Protector Within is concerned about safety at all times. This means that the human mind is very threat-focused and at times can be overly critical and protective. You learned in previous chapters that the human mind is concerned with safety, protection and threats of danger. Sometimes your mind will tell you things that are not entirely helpful. When you automatically listen to your thoughts and see the world through those thoughts, it can drive your behavior. When this happens, it can move you away from the life you want and the things that are important to you. It is like looking at life from behind a waterfall of thoughts that are overly critical, judgmental and threat-focused.

When you see the world through your thoughts, rather than from your thoughts, it can restrict your view and the choices you make. Learning to look at thoughts from a different perspective can help you decide if they are helpful or not, depending on the given situation.

Special Hearing Aids

For the next 30 seconds, imagine you are wearing a very special pair of hearing aids that allow you to listen to what your mind is saying.

- Notice the flow of thoughts and all the different topics that come up. Allow yourself to get lost in them for 30 seconds to one minute.
- Notice one thought your mind is having and name it; "I'm thinking about_____
_____."

- Notice if your mind switches topics.
- Notice if the content of your thinking changes from happy to sad, or fearful to brave, or engaged to bored.
- Notice if thoughts stop momentarily. Just keep listening until they start again.

There is a part of your mind that does all the thinking and talking. This perspective can help you gain some distance from your thoughts and the impact they are having on your life. If you are too close, it can be hard to notice thoughts, especially when they are quickly racing by. The following exercise will help you step back from your thoughts even further.

 Noticing Thoughts as Thoughts

- Take a moment to identify one thought about pain.
  - It could be a worry you have about pain, a fear about pain, or an evaluative judgment about its cause. *For example, "The cartilage in my knee is worn out."*
- Continue to think this thought for 30 seconds, slowly repeating it over and over with some degree of conviction.
  - Do you notice any physical sensations develop as a result of that thought?
  - Do you notice any emotions that show up?
- Continue to simply allow this thought to be present for another 30 seconds.
- Now, repeat the thought and in front of it place the phrase, "I'm having the thought that
_____
_____."

For example, "I'm having the thought that the cartilage in my knee is worn out."
Repeat this a few times.
  - Do you notice anything?
- Now, let's add to this and in front of it place the phrase, "I'm noticing that I'm having the thought that _____
_____."

For example, "I'm noticing that I'm having the thought that the cartilage in my knee is worn out."
Repeat this a few times.
- Finally, let's add a third piece to the sentence and in front of it place the phrase, "I'm noticing that I'm thinking about having the thought that _____
_____."

For example, "I'm noticing that I'm thinking about having the thought that the cartilage in my knee is worn out." Repeat this a few times.
  - What did you notice?

There is a part of your mind that does the talking, and you can notice what thoughts it is sending downstream. Sometimes it's just a trickle and other times it's a deluge. If your mind is like my mind and the billions of other minds on the planet, we have very little control over what thoughts are being generated. To date, modern science hasn't figured out a way to slow down, shut off or control thoughts. That's the stuff of science fiction. However, we do have the ability to become more aware of our thinking and learn how to respond differently.

Notice what your mind is telling you right now at this very moment. What would happen if you allowed yourself to follow through with that thought or get caught up in the thought? Have you considered that if you buy into every thought your mind serves up about pain, it may pull you away from overcoming it? Please don't be overly critical—your mind is simply doing what it evolved to do. As you practice and learn to watch your thoughts non-judgmentally, you can gently thank your mind for its amazing ability to think. An active mind is important. But if you can notice your thoughts for what they are, and not what they say they are, you can choose to act on those thoughts, or not to act, if it helps you live a better life. Try this exercise for more practice.

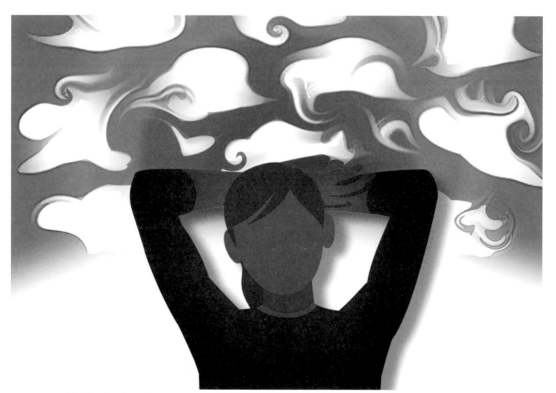

Noticing thoughts and allowing them to float away like clouds gives you space to decide how you want to react.

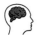 **Watching Thoughts Float By**

First, find a comfortable position seated in a chair. Sit upright with your feet flat on the floor, your arms and legs uncrossed, and your hands resting on your lap. Allow your eyes to close or fix them on a point in front of you.

- Take five gentle breaths in and out.
- Notice the sensation of your own breath as you breathe in and out. Now, imagine you are lying in a grassy field on a warm summer day.
- Notice feeling the ground beneath you, the smell of the grass, and the sounds of nearby trees blowing in the wind.
- Now, imagine you are looking up at the sky, watching clouds pass by.
- Start to become conscious of your thoughts.
- Each time a thought pops into your head, imagine placing it on one of these clouds and allow it to float on by.
- If you think in words or images, place these on a cloud, and let them float by.
- Continue watching the sky and allow the clouds to keep moving by. Try not to change what shows up on the clouds in any way. If the clouds disappear or you go somewhere else mentally, simply stop and notice this happening, and gently bring yourself back to watching the clouds in the sky.
- If you have any thoughts about doing this exercise, place these on the clouds, as well.
- If your thoughts stop, simply watch the sky and the clouds. Eventually your thoughts will start up again.
- You are simply observing each thought as a word or an image on a cloud.
- Let the clouds float on by at their own pace and place any thought that comes to mind on a cloud and allow it to float on by.
- Finally, bring your attention back to your breathing. Notice again the steady rhythm of your breath that is with you all the time.
- Then, bring your awareness back to the present moment. Gently open your eyes and notice what you see. Push your feet into the floor and stretch; notice yourself stretching.

How did you do with this exercise? What was it like noticing thoughts rather than getting carried away by thinking them? The only goal of this exercise is to notice the process of thinking, nothing more. Not to slow thoughts, speed them up or make them go away. Once you start watching thoughts it can be fascinating how fast they come and go, how some are dark and stormy, and others are bright and sunny. You may have been present in the moment noticing thoughts for a while and then minutes later woke up from having drifted off into a story about the future or replaying the past.

> Our minds are very good at hooking us into thinking about our thoughts rather than seeing them for what they are—just thoughts. Most of us assume that we need to change thoughts we don't like or that cause us distress. Changing thoughts doesn't work so well and can cause us to suffer more. Now you have to change pain and change thoughts. Now you have to control pain and control thoughts about pain. Becoming curious while you watch and listen to thoughts can help you develop a sense of distance from them. By watching and naming thoughts you create space between the thought, and it gives you an opportunity to decide how you will react. This is helpful—it provides you with room to respond and an opportunity to move toward who and what you really care about.

CHAPTER 12: UNHOOKING FROM THOUGHTS

It is common to attempt to avoid, change, or push away unpleasant thoughts, emotions, memories or bodily sensations. This process is called "avoidance" and it prevents us from living life to the fullest. When we get "hooked" by thoughts it's as though they push us around or bully us, like a critical coach standing on the sidelines, giving negative feedback such as, "that was stupid," "you're weak," or, "you can't do that if you're in pain." The mind is like a thought-generating machine, and your thoughts can be like hooks. What happens when you get hooked?

Learning to become more aware of our thinking and observing thoughts without judging, evaluating or trying to change them is one way to move beyond pain. This process teaches you to pay attention to the experience of having thoughts, rather than focusing on their meaning (i.e., there must be something wrong with me). This doesn't mean that you have to like or want the thought. It is about acknowledging that you are having the thought and that attempts to push it away or struggling with it may not be helpful. Consider your own experience with thoughts: Has trying to change, avoid or distract from thoughts worked for you? Or, if it works sometimes does it work in the long run? For example, have you noticed that when you try not to think about something (or someone) you end up thinking more about it? Try the next exercise to help you understand how difficult it is to stop thoughts.

 ### Elephants, Elephants, Elephants

Take out a stopwatch or use the timer on your smartphone. For the next three minutes, do not think about pink elephants. As you watch the timer tick down, do whatever you have to do to keep yourself from thinking about pink elephants. You can think about other things—baseball, the most recent movie you saw, your sister or brother, just don't think about pink elephants. Should you think about a pink elephant, note how many times the pink elephant comes to mind. Begin now.

How many times did you think about pink elephants during the exercise? One time, five times, ten times? If you are like most people, pink elephants kept showing up—even if you tried to put them out of your mind or distract yourself. Distraction may help for a few minutes, maybe even an hour, but does it make the thoughts and feelings go away in the long term?

It's possible to build up your willingness to have unwanted thoughts by practicing a few simple techniques that help you develop greater awareness. Just as you can do physical exercise to build muscles in your body, you can do mental exercises to develop mental "muscle," allowing you to increase your awareness.

Key skills can be learned to help you let go of the struggle to control unwanted thoughts. This can help you focus on the here and now and more fully engage in the present moment. This is helpful because, through thinking, our minds have the ability to time travel. Thoughts can pull you into the future and often cause anxiety, or to dwell on the past and cause depression. Focusing on the present moment and acting in ways that are consistent with your values can keep you centered.

Rather than trying to get rid of anxious or fearful thoughts, you can shift your focus. Imagine focusing your energy on what really matters in your life, by setting and working toward your goals and dreams. For example, a new mom may feel anxious and scared about low back pain preventing her from doing what's most important to her—taking care of her newborn daughter. Even though thoughts about pain may arise, she can decide she is going to do the things she needs to do, even with these thoughts. Thoughts can come along for the ride and not influence her behavior. After all, if she waits until she is completely pain-free before doing all she can to be the mom she wants to be, she may be waiting a very long time before she can care for her daughter and fulfill her dream of being a mom.

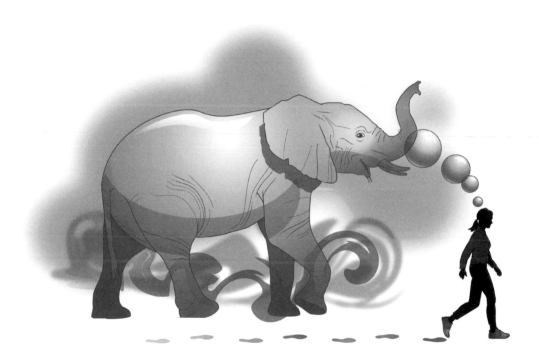

Trying not to think about a pink elephant will likely cause you to think about one thing: a pink elephant.

Learning to let thoughts be without having to change or get rid of your inner dialogue, feelings and physical sensations can be challenging and you will need some time to practice. As an exercise to build awareness, write down three thoughts about pain that often hook you (in the clouds below).

Now, hold the paper up at arm's length in front of you and read the three thoughts you wrote on the clouds. Does anything change? Now prop it up on the table or tape it to a wall and step back from it as far as you can while still being able to read it. Does stepping back 5, 10 or 20 feet change the stickiness of these thoughts? Do the thoughts feel like they are less a part of you now that you've gained some physical distance from them? Does your relationship to the thoughts change? Have your thoughts lost some of their truth, influence or power? Can you read and be with these thoughts while you do something with your body such as balancing on one foot or gently dancing in place? If you are like most people, writing distressing thoughts down and stepping back from them helps change their influence on how you feel and act.

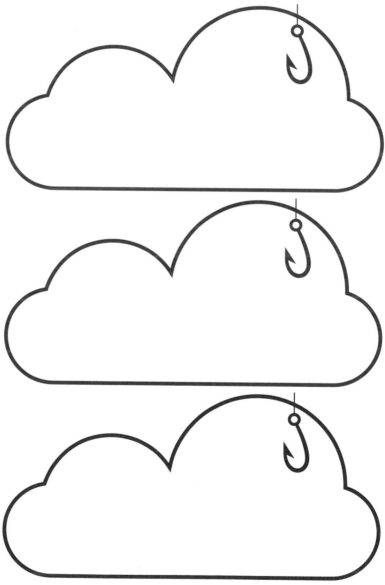

It's possible to unhook yourself from your thoughts and allow them to float away like clouds.

CHAPTER 13: THE SECOND ARROW

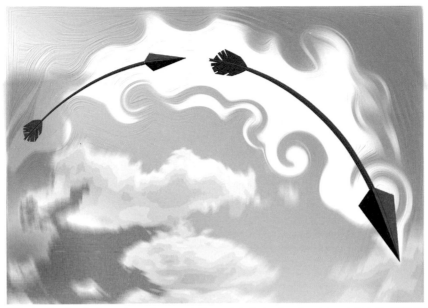

Buddhism teaches that the "second arrow" represents the psychological and emotional struggle that often follows pain.

The most current scientific explanation of pain describes it as both a physical and emotional experience. In fact, an observation of the brain in pain under a high-tech functional MRI shows areas light up as bright as the constellation Orion. Some of these areas represent physical body parts. Interestingly, the emotional centers light up as well and areas related to thoughts and emotions often shine the brightest.

It is a fact of life that humans don't like pain. We almost always work to avoid pain and seek effective measures of pain control. If we can't find satisfactory relief we struggle and resist it. How can a person live a full life when chronic pain is present, with both physical and emotional effects?

The effect that pain has on humans, both physically and emotionally, supports Buddhist teachings from centuries ago—long before our modern methods existed. The Buddhists called it the "second arrow." The Buddha taught physical pain is like being shot with a single arrow—it pierces the skin and hurts. The person who does not resist physical pain feels only the

arrow. However, all humans—by the nature of our thinking and problem-solving minds—add on a layer of psychological and emotional struggle. We think about, ruminate and anguish over pain. This is like being shot by an extremely sharp second arrow that penetrates deeply into the skin.

Although we commonly experience physical pain as a single sensation, it is actually composed of multiple elements, including an avoidance element we call suffering. Not only does avoidance create suffering—the second arrow—it's increasingly clear that our response to pain can affect the first arrow, the pain sensation itself. Once we experience pain we rally all of our attention around it. Simply bringing attention (and especially fearful attention) to pain, increases the experience of pain. Pain is perpetuated by fear, worry, anxiety and every unpleasant emotion known to man. Avoidance causes suffering, which causes more pain, which causes more suffering. Ancient wisdom has influenced modern-day pain care and helps us understand pain.

Recognizing Clean Pain and Dirty Pain

In ACT we have a similar approach to the second arrow effect, and it's one that has helped many people become aware of the difference between physical pain and the emotional and behavioral responses that often follow. This approach includes two types of pain—*clean pain and dirty pain*. Clean pain is the description you make of the physical pain—the pain you felt. Dirty pain includes the reactions you have to the pain—including what you think or do in response. By tuning in and becoming aware of your thoughts, emotions and reactions you can change the way you respond to pain, and more importantly, change the amount of suffering you experience. The exercise below can help you recognize the difference between clean pain and dirty pain and the effect it has on pain intensity. Here are a few real-life events and the distinction between clean pain and dirty pain.

| Event | Clean Pain | | Dirty Pain | |
	What is the sensation you feel?	Pain Intensity	What do you think or do in response?	Pain Intensity
Scrubbed and cleaned both bathrooms in my house.	Sharp pain on the right side of my back and into my right buttock.	6	Started wondering if I herniated the disc more in my back and how I'll never be able to care for myself or my family.	9
Drove 2 hours to my sister's house.	Building stiffness and tension in my neck and upper shoulders.	5	That day lost my temper and became very angry at my sister for not coming to visit me when she knows I have pain, which turned into an argument about her lack of involvement and support in caring for our elderly mother.	10
Had a session with a substitute Pilates instructor because my usual instructor was out sick.	Had increased SI joint pain and muscle spasms in my lower back.	7	The instructor didn't understand my needs and pushed me too hard. Went straight home, stayed on the couch all day and then went to bed early. Popped a pain killer before bed.	8

Use the chart below to fill in how events in your life impact your clean pain and dirty pain, and how dirty pain affects the activities that are important in your life.

| Event | Clean Pain | | Dirty Pain | |
	What is the sensation you feel?	Pain Intensity	What do you think or do in response?	Pain Intensity

Being present with, turning toward, and saying "yes" to the unpleasant sensations is one path out of suffering. We suffer because we marry our instinctive avoidance patterns to the deep-seated belief that life should be free from all pain. In resisting pain and by holding this belief, we strengthen that which we're trying to avoid. When we make pain the enemy, we engage in the struggle and solidify it as a constant thorn in our side. Noticing our own natural avoidance, resistance and, most importantly, how we suffer, is one path toward living fully.

CHAPTER 14: WORDS THAT HURT

If you watch a professional dancer perform, you will notice how they are completely present in the moment. Some call this a "flow" state, also known as being in the "zone." Being in a state of flow, or in the zone, is a mental state in which a person is fully immersed in a feeling of focus, full involvement, and enjoyment in the process of the activity they are performing. Attention becomes so centered on the task at hand that everything else disappears. Action and awareness merge and sense of self vanishes. Time becomes relative. During this moment, all aspects of performance (both mental and physical) are improved. Movement is unencumbered by thoughts.

A dancer performing while in pain can result in a very different experience. When pain is present the mind redirects attention on pain. The awareness that dissolved time and space is likely to be interrupted by the intrusion of thought. As the choreography is played out in the mind, attention is drawn to protection, instead of peak performance. When asked to describe pain, dancers and other people living with pain use elaborate language to describe their experience. The mind creates thoughts in the form of words and images in an attempt to make sense and solve the problem. Sharp pain requires we dull it. Burning pain sounds the alarm to put out the fire. If it is radiating, let's reel it in or centralize it. Feeling tight and tense? Stretch it, so it feels loose and relaxed. If tender, then we must strengthen. Words seem to have a solution to our pain.

However, if you take a moment to create some distance and space, you'll begin to notice that thoughts are simply words, not concrete tangible objects. This will help open your mind to more than the automatic conclusions and reactions you may draw from those words. The next exercise will help you to understand that thoughts are just words.

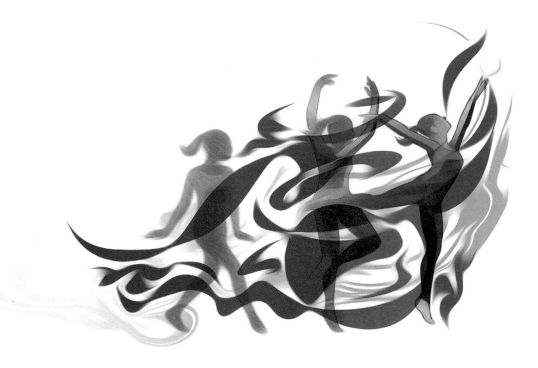

Dancers often experience a state of flow that brings a feeling of focus, full involvement and enjoyment in the process.

Playing with Thoughts

In this exercise, think of all the qualities associated with the word "milk." Think of its pale white color. Think of the smell of milk and its rich, creamy taste. Now repeat the word "milk" over and over again as fast as you can for 45 seconds. Most people find that the word eventually loses all associations, becoming a series of meaningless sounds or vocalizations.

Now, repeat the exercise using a thought you tell yourself when you're experiencing pain or when you're afraid of getting hurt. Choose a word or phrase with a strong negative quality like "weak," "damaged," "broken," "bad knee," or "back pain." You can use more judgmental words like "weakling," or "useless," but don't use these harsh words the first time around. Now say the word out loud as fast as you can for 45 seconds.

Now, with your eyes closed imagine you can see this word on a computer screen. Once you have this image in your mind, see if you can change the colors of the letters. Then change the font of the letters. Now, mix and match the fonts and the colors of the letters. Finally, see if you can make the letters move and dance around on the screen.

Stop and notice—does the word still sound as valid and believable as it once did? Did you notice how the word started to lose some of its significance and influence? Similar to the word "milk," negative words begin to lose their meaning when spoken repeatedly. If you think in images they also begin to lose their significance when you see or picture them differently. Pause a few times today to notice your thoughts. Then try the above exercise. Notice if the meaning of the word changes or if you begin to feel some separation from thoughts. You are not your thoughts, nor your feelings, sensations or memories.

CHAPTER 15: VOICES OF PAIN

Place your hand over your heart and notice how it beats. Continue this for one minute, noticing the thump and constant rhythm of your heart. At an average of 80 beats per minute, your heart beats about 4,800 times per hour. That's a whopping 115,200 times per day!

While it beats, your heart circulates nutrients to all your organs. Just as your heart continues to beat, beat, beat, your mind continues to think, think, think, all day long. The human mind is like a thought-generating machine. Neuroscientists estimate that the mind thinks an average of 2,500 – 3,300 thoughts per hour. That's between 60,000 – 80,000 thoughts a day! Your mind is very active doing what it does best, thinking. That's what minds do. Unlike your heart, you can't place your hand on your head and feel thinking. You have to use certain exercises to develop an awareness of your thoughts so that you know what your mind is broadcasting.

In previous chapters, we talked about the Protector Within—a part of you that takes on a personality of its own and is trying to protect you. The Protector Within is concerned with a few very important things such as food, water, shelter, and even sex. But most importantly, the Protector is concerned about your safety. To the Protector, safety never takes a holiday! One important job of the Protector is to predict when and where you might get hurt. It does this by broadcasting thoughts, commands, and rules about potential and actual pain. However, not every thought the Protector broadcasts is helpful or even necessary. And when it comes to chronic pain, the Protector often gets it wrong.

But, the Protector Within wants to be heard. At times it may seem like the voice of the Protector Within drones on in the background, and at other times he may be yelling at you. His voice, words, and predictions come from the belief that pain equals damage, that you are hurting yourself, and that it's impossible to feel pain and still live a full life. The Protector Within keeps you focused on eliminating and controlling pain as the way out of suffering.

The voice of the Protector is constantly broadcasting the rule that pain must be completely gone before you can return to an active life. It lays down the law that pain relief comes first, then your life. To break free from this cycle, it's useful to notice when the Protector is voicing an unhelpful solution. The next exercise can help.

Noticing Unhelpful Thoughts about Pain

Use the worksheet below to explore some of your thoughts about pain. Write down any thought about pain that comes to mind. Below are eight common areas people tend to think and worry about when it comes to their pain. Your thoughts influence the things you do. Below are some examples of how thoughts can influence our behavior and cause us to suffer. Use this to keep a record of what you do when painful thoughts arise and notice if these actions lead to increased vitality or increased suffering.

What the Protector Thinks	What Your Thoughts Lead To
Thoughts about pain and damage	
I think pain means something is broken.	Stay home, don't move, and don't do anything that causes pain.
I think pain means something is not working.	Go to another "specialist" to find the cause.
Thoughts about pain and exercise	
Exercise makes the pain worse.	Only exercise when I'm 100% pain-free. Otherwise rest and stay on the couch.
Exercise is for people without pain.	Eliminate the pain first, then start exercising.
Thoughts about pain and work	
Work is where I hurt myself.	If I go back to work I'll hurt myself. Call in sick and stay home.
If I complain about pain at work I'll get fired.	White knuckling and pushing through pain.
Thoughts about controlling pain	
I can't leave home without my pills.	I need my pills to survive. Carry them everywhere.
Thoughts about pain and sleep	
It's going to be another night of tossing and turning!	Think all night about my pain and how it's going to destroy the next day.
I wonder if the pain will wake me up again?	Have a drink or two before bed.
Thoughts about pain and relationships	
I can't go out and see my friends because I have pain.	Don't make plans to see friends until the pain is gone!
I can't be intimate with my husband.	Don't get too close to people, they will expect too much from me.
Thoughts about pain and my health	
I think pain means I'm weak and fragile.	Feeling helpless and hopeless.
Thoughts about pain and my future	
I can't make plans because I'll never know if the pain will start.	Don't plan for the future, its unknown!
I feel I can't go on.	Go back to bed.

Fill in the blanks with your thoughts about pain and what actions they often lead to.

Thoughts	What Your Thoughts Lead To
Thoughts about pain and damage	
Thoughts about pain and exercise	
Thoughts about pain and work	
Thoughts about controlling pain	
Thoughts about pain and sleep	
Thoughts about pain and relationships	
Thoughts about pain and my health	
Thoughts about pain and my future	

CHAPTER 16: THE PAIN CHAIN

Previous chapters provided the opportunity for you to begin building essential skills to help you notice thoughts and gain some distance from them. You also learned that imbedded in what we identify as pain are thoughts about pain and how those thoughts can lead to further suffering.

This chapter continues to build on these concepts by showing how your thoughts can cause a chain reaction in your life. They can be a catalyst that can spark extraordinary results and outcomes. In an earlier chapter, you learned how the second arrow of dirty pain can be used to ease the suffering around pain. The next exercise will show you how dirty pain can be the first domino to fall, causing a series of chain reactions.

 Identifying the Chain

The first step is to identify an event that causes pain. It can be an actual event, like cleaning the house or exercising, or it can be just thinking about doing something. Next, notice the dirty pain or the distressing thought the mind produces in response to the event. Third, based on your thoughts, what type of action did you take? It could be an action you took to control or eliminate pain or something you avoided doing to prevent further pain. Last, write the name of someone who you missed seeing, or something you skipped doing when you followed the advice of your thoughts. A few examples are provided below.

Event That Caused Pain	Thoughts About Pain	Action Based on Thoughts	Who or What You Skipped/Missed
Woke up with back pain	The disc must be pressing on the nerve.	Sat on couch with hot pack and called in sick.	Work Financially supporting my family. Happy hour with work friends.
Lifting groceries at store	I need another steroid injection.	Couldn't complete grocery shopping. Sat in car and cried for 10-minutes. Drove home, called the doctor and then called for pizza delivery. Overindulged on food.	Healthy meals Supporting my family's health. Being a capable mother and wife. Nurturing my body and weight.
Long day sitting at work	Sitting is damaging my spine. If I have pain then I can't work.	Got home and took painkiller. Watched TV and fell asleep on couch.	Talking with my husband when he got home from work. Helping my daughter with her homework.

Now it's your turn. Fill in the spaces below.

Event That Caused Pain	Thoughts About Pain	Action Based on Thoughts	Who or What You Skipped/Missed

Like a string of dominos, this chain reaction can happen in reverse or even start in the middle. Most often it is an event that leads to distressing thoughts about pain, which can lead to controlling or avoiding pain, instead of living your life. These small chain reactions can quickly balloon into large problems as habits form and you begin to miss out on important parts of your life. The growth and impact of dirty pain can be exponential if left unchecked. You may not notice how your thoughts have taken over the wheel steering you in unwanted directions. Noticing gives you the opportunity to make different choices, allowing you to start taking back control of your life.

CHAPTER 17: THE STORYTELLING MIND

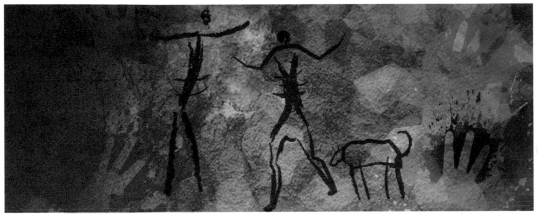

Storytelling is central to human evolution and serves as a way to educate, nurture and support.

Anthropologists tell us that storytelling is central to human evolution. Storytelling is common to every known culture and has existed in many forms. Stories involve an exchange between the storyteller and listener— an exchange we learn from a very young age. Stories are told around campfires, on the radio and through all forms of media. They serve as a way to educate, nurture and support. Stories include recognizable patterns, and in those patterns we find meaning. We use stories to make sense of our world and to share that understanding with others. So powerful is our impulse to detect stories that we sometimes create stories even when they're not there.

Our minds evolved to be great storytellers. Many of the stories our minds tell are crafted to keep us out of harm's way and prevent pain. The mind is never short of a story to tell, and it yearns for us to listen, whatever the story is. Like any great storyteller, the mind will say whatever it has to say to get our attention. Some stories are true: we can call these facts. Others are opinions, beliefs, ideas, assumptions or predictions. Just listen now, to the story your mind is telling you.

Some stories broadcast doom and gloom about the past, future or present. It is like a staticky old transistor radio blaring in the background that can't be ignored. Other stories cast a main character that makes all sorts of demands, a spoiled brat that throws tantrums if it doesn't get its own way. He will kick and scream until you give in. Some stories have the leading man take on the role of a fascist dictator constantly ordering you about and telling you what you can and can't do.

Like a Hollywood screenwriter, your mind is always writing the next story. If you simply ask yourself, "Who am I?" your mind will come up with all sorts of self-descriptions, quickly filling in the blank. "I am a _____
_____."

This could be, "I am a woman," "I am a wife," "I am someone with fibromyalgia," or, "I am a chronic pain patient."

Sometimes the responses are beautifully scripted one-liners and other times they are elaborate accounts about the person you are today. The mind writes many stories and the more absorbed you become, the more you get hooked into the stories your mind is telling. You are cut off from everything except the ongoing storyline. It's like being stuck in a loop watching a Netflix series that never ends, keeping you glued to the couch, unable to get out to enjoy life. The word machine of the mind churns out a never-ending stream of thoughts, crafted into a story that may list reasons why you can't or shouldn't change. Because we are so close to our own thoughts, we believe everything the mind says is very important and we must pay attention. But we do have a choice. We can choose to notice the story and unhook from it.

We can choose to watch the show our mind is playing from a distance, without getting up on stage and performing. We can be observers, versus actors inside the play.

 ## Watch the Show

Find a comfortable seated position with your feet on the floor. You can either close your eyes or fix them on a spot about two feet in front of you.

- Take a few moments and notice how you are breathing. Count at least five in-and-out breaths.
- Then take a few moments to notice what you see. Notice what you hear. Notice what you smell or taste. Notice your thoughts. Notice what you are feeling. Notice what you are doing.
- A part of you is doing all the noticing. Noticing everything you see, hear, taste, smell, feel and think. We call this the "observing self" or the "observer." This part of you is always present doing all the noticing. The observing self is the part of you that can step back and watch the stage show. On that stage are all of your thoughts, feelings and everything you can see, hear, taste and smell. You can step back and take it all in or you can zoom in on any one aspect.
- Now return to your breath. Notice how your abdomen rises and falls. Take 10 nice, easy in-and-out breaths.
- Notice how during this time the mind began to think and tell stories. The masterful storyteller in the mind doesn't allow us to be idle for long before it begins to tap you on the shoulder and pull your attention away from the present moment and what you are doing.
- See if you can let your mind chatter in the background like a news reporter on the radio. Don't try and turn the radio off or adjust the volume; that can't be done. Just allow the mind to broadcast whatever story it's playing. Keep your attention on your breath as it plays.
- Notice any feelings or sensations that arise in the body. You may feel bored, tired, anxious or frustrated. You may have some back pain, knee pain or tension in your neck and shoulders. The mind will chatter away and create a story around that, too.
- Life is like a stage show, and on that stage are all of your thoughts, feelings and everything you can see, hear, taste, smell and touch. In this exercise, you directed the spotlight on one aspect of your body, the breath.
- Now shine the spotlight on other parts of your body. Notice your arms, legs, feet, hands and torso.
- Notice you are in a room; look around at what you see, hear, smell, taste and touch.
- There's a part of you inside that can notice everything.
- Last, notice what you are thinking.

You are the author of your story. We all tell stories to make sense of our lives. Despite what's been written so far, what do you want your life to be about? The mind creates stories to try and explain what is happening and protect us from future harm. Stories in and of themselves are harmless, unless you buy into them. The problem is we listen to our own stories about ourselves. When this happens, we believe the stories and get wrapped up in the plot. Stories about who we are and what we are capable of can contain us. It can be unpleasant to look at our stories because they seemingly have promised to keep us safe. Noticing our stories can help us drop them and open up an opportunity for us to actively rewrite the script of our own lives.

CHAPTER 18: MOVING WITH THE MIND

Mindful movement is the act of engaging in an exercise or activity performed with awareness. It involves mental focus to train your body to move optimally. Mindful movement combines deep breathing and controlled movement with an open focus guided by intention. While it may sound complicated, mindful movement is anything but hard to understand. Put simply, it refers to engaging in physical activity while placing your attention and awareness on the movement of your body while alternately noticing your environment.

Movement and activity are more than just physical. When performed mindfully, they allow the mind to focus, engage and be present. The breath supports movement, and your awareness and attention helps you feel and appreciate the subtleties of actions. Moving mindfully is an effective way to get the most out of your physical activity and can lower stress, anxiety and fear associated with pain.

When a person experiences pain, the mind places it under the microscope for investigation. The mind and the body become narrowly focused on pain. This *narrow focus of attention* is stressful and causes the breath to become shallow and rapid, blood vessels constrict, and pressure rises, the digestive system shuts down, muscles and the mind fatigue and psychological distress increases. A mindful and *open focus of attention*, on the other hand, is the opposite. An open focus is a relaxed state complemented by an awareness of the environment.

There are five principles of mindful movement with an open focus.

1. **Breathing:** All movement is performed with the rhythm of the breath. This may be achieved during one specific exercise or continually as you engage in normal daily activities.

2. **Centering:** The process of focusing and refocusing on the breath center, the spot just below your belly button. This is a place to anchor and defuse from the minds process of thinking and the bodies sensation making.

3. **Concentration:** Movement is executed with full concentration. Attention is placed on the movement or exercise in order to obtain maximum value and benefit. The mind is centered as the body moves through space.

4. **Control:** Every exercise or movement is performed with complete intention and control. No body part is left to its own devices. It is conscious and deliberate movement.

5. **Precision:** A heightened state of awareness is sustained throughout each movement. There is an appropriate placement relative to other body parts and quality of movement is improved.

Mindful movement also offers another important benefit. It provides you with a method of exposing yourself to potentially distressing situations as you increase activity. Like an Olympic figure skater, you will learn to glide over soft edges that seem safe and secure as well as hard edges that elicit fear and anxiety. This helps you increase your physical activity even when movement seems uncertain, your mind tells you otherwise or the Protector Within begins to spin.

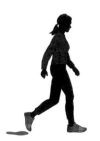

There is an important distinction to make before we move further. It is a myth that the mind controls our movement and actions. The mind does not control our movement. We control our movement. As you learned earlier, the mind is always thinking, judging and problem-solving, and the Protector Within goes into high alert as we aim to increase physical activity. For example, I can be performing a relatively simple exercise and notice my mind chattering away in the background saying things like "this exercise is not good for my back," "this is too difficult," or "stop before you hurt yourself." We can allow our mind to think as we move anyway. You can move and take your mind along for the ride.

It is like driving a bus while the passengers in the back start threatening you, telling you what you have to do and where you have to go. Some of them are yelling at you and others are scary, dressed in black leather jackets and carrying switchblade knives. You are scared that if you don't do what they say they will come up from the back of the bus and take over. So, in order to solve the problem and rid yourself of these noisy passengers you kick them off the bus. You stop the bus and go back to deal with the aggressive passengers. But you notice that the very first thing you had to do was stop. Notice now, you're not driving anywhere, you're just dealing with the passengers. And these passengers are smart as they get right back on at the next stop.

In other words, by trying to get control, you've actually given up control! Now notice that even though your passengers claim they can tell you what to do and hurt you if you don't turn left, it has never actually happened. These passengers can't make you do something against your will. Which passenger is threatening you now? Who's doing the driving? Your body is the bus and you are the driver. The noisy passengers in the back are like your thoughts, feelings, memories and bodily sensations. You can steer the bus in the direction you want to go and do the opposite of what your mind is telling you. To demonstrate that thoughts do not control your behavior or movement, complete the following activities.

 Do the Opposite

Think to yourself, "I can't scratch my chin! I can't scratch my chin!" And as you do, lift your arm and scratch your chin.

Think to yourself, "I have to stand up! I have to stand up!" And as you do that, stay seated.

Now say aloud, "I can't raise my right arm! I can't raise my right arm!" And as you do that, raise your right arm as high as you can.

How did you do? Were you able to do the opposite despite the command not to do something? No doubt you found that you could perform those actions even though your mind and thoughts said you couldn't. Of course, thoughts can influence your behavior—but they can't control it. As you begin to become more physically active, the mind will offer new reasons why you shouldn't move and create more stories. Who is in charge of your body? You or your mind? If we fuse with our thoughts, it will have a greater influence on our behavior and movement.

The reasons our mind offers are not a problem unless we fuse with them; that is, take them as the literal truth, or treat them as commands we must obey. It's important to realize that reasons are not facts. Here's an example of a reason: "I can't go for a walk because I'm too tired, and I hurt." But does being tired and having some pain make you physically unable to walk? In most instances, no. You can feel tired, have pain and still go for a walk. In fact, ask any physical therapist and they'll tell you that we help people walk right after hip and knee replacements, even when they are feeling tired and have pain. Walking is the therapy to decrease pain and increase stamina. Continue to explore mindful movement with the next exercise.

 ## Mindful Walking

Set aside five minutes for this next exercise and find a place where you can walk with relatively few interruptions. Options may be around your backyard, neighborhood or the high school track.

As you walk, first bring your awareness to your mind. Listen to what you mind is saying. Notice and name one thought such as, "I'm thinking about _____

_____."

As you walk, simply notice the flow of your thoughts. Stay with this for a minute as you walk.

Next, shift the focus of your attention to your breath center. See if you can feel from which part on the front of your body you are breathing. Do you notice your breath in your chest or more down toward your belly button? See if you can stay with your breath for one minute. If your focus shifts to the chattering of the mind, thank your mind for thinking, and then gently refocus on the breath center. Stay with this for a minute.

Then, shift the focus of your attention to your body. Scan your body for one physical sensation other than the breath. It may be muscles contracting, your heart beating or the feeling of the ground beneath your feet. As you connect to this sensation see if you can shift the focus back to your breath, then to what your mind is saying, and then back again to a sensation in your body. Play with this shifting focus for a minute.

Now, speed up and walk faster and with more intention. Increase your strides and allow the arms to swing. Notice what the mind does and watch your thinking. Does it start to give you reasons why you shouldn't speed up or demand that you slow down? Become aware of how the breath increases and physical sensations in the body change. How does this increased velocity make you feel? Is there a particular emotion that presents itself? Commit to walking briskly and stay with this for a minute and observe all the changes that occur.

Finally, see if you can connect to why this activity is important. Do you have friends you miss and would enjoy traveling with (which requires you to be on your feet)? Do you have a husband who needs a supportive workout partner to help him lose a few pounds? Have you dreamed of accompanying your granddaughter on her school trips, which require stamina? As you are walking, breathing, and thinking, connect to one reason why this is important. Stay with this for a minute.

You can apply the principles of mindful walking to any activity. Begin with an activity that is easy to gain practice and later move on to exercises or physical activities that cause some fear or anxiety.

Mindful movement integrates the three parts of each one of us—mind, heart and body. This is the work of thinking, feeling and moving. When all three parts of our cognitive, emotional and kinesthetic abilities are toned it is more effective for pain than static or sedentary mindfulness.

Mindful movement occurs when an awareness of the present moment is guided by the rhythm of the breath. It entails you watch your thinking, embraces a variety of bodily sensations, occurs in changing contexts, requires a commitment to moving in and out hard edges, and is linked to things in life that bring you joy, meaning and purpose.

CHAPTER 19: BREAKING FREE

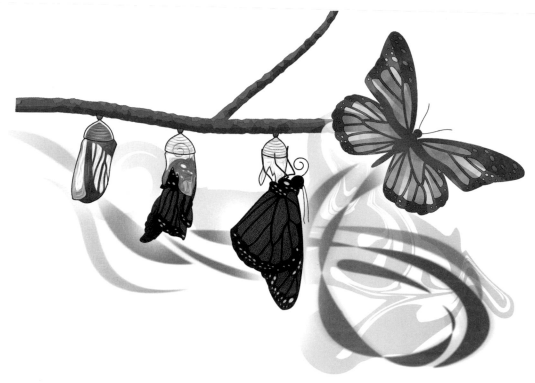

A butterfly's struggle to emerge from the cocoon helps it gain the strength it needs to fly.

One day a man walking on a wooded trail came across a Monarch butterfly cocoon. He was familiar with the beauty of the Monarch and the way it calmly sailed through the air. He was so enthralled with the butterfly that he decided to take it home so he could watch it grow and emerge from its cocoon. To his excitement, one day, a small opening appeared in the cocoon. He poured a cup of tea and sat quietly, watching the butterfly for several hours as it struggled to force its body through the hole. Suddenly, the little butterfly stopped moving. It appeared to have gotten as far as it could and now seemed stuck.

Out of kindness, the man decided to help the butterfly break free. He took a pair of scissors and snipped away at the remaining parts of the cocoon. The butterfly emerged from the cocoon, but to the man's dismay, the butterfly's body was swollen and its tiny wings were shriveled. The man continued to watch, hoping that at any moment the wings would enlarge and unfold, fully able to support the body of the butterfly. Neither happened; The little butterfly spent the rest of its life crawling around with a swollen body and shriveled wings. It never was able to fly.

For the butterfly to complete the metamorphosis from caterpillar to a beautiful winged Monarch and safely emerge from its cocoon, it needed to experience the painful struggle of change and break free on its own from the temporary safety of the restricting cocoon. It was a necessary part of the metamorphosis process; to grow and force fluid from the body and into the wings so the butterfly would be ready for flight once it emerged. Freedom and flight would only come after a difficult and painful struggle.

Mother nature instinctively knows what to do. Humans share this wisdom with all creatures, but sometimes our thinking minds can get in the way. It is not easy to overcome pain when thoughts, feelings, physical sensations and memories show up and become intense. These negative thoughts and feelings can drain away any hope and pull you from what's important.

The urge to control pain and the yearning for complete relief can be just as intense as the pain itself. It can cause you to retreat into the safety of your cocoon or make you want to speed up the process. You can learn to redirect these yearnings toward your life values. The next two exercises will teach you how to hold thoughts and other inner sensations lightly and to open up to the full experience of overcoming pain.

Holding Thoughts Lightly

Begin by spending a few minutes with your eyes closed, breathing deeply.

Now imagine yourself sitting in a field on a warm summer day. Take a few moments to visualize yourself in this place. Imagine the feeling of the warm sun on your face and a slight breeze on your skin. Smell the grass and imagine the flowers gently moving in the breeze. Your breath is your anchor.

- As you connect with this experience, your thoughts may start to wander. Imagine these wandering thoughts as a steady stream of butterflies flying past you.
- As you notice your thoughts as butterflies, observe the wide variety of butterflies. Some may look familiar, comforting and attractive, while others are unappealing and may even make you feel uneasy.
- Notice how you are drawn to the pleasant and familiar butterflies while avoiding or pushing away the unpleasant and unappealing ones.
- To embody this experience, take your right hand and hold it out with your palm open, allowing the pleasant butterflies to land on your hand. Then, with your left hand, begin swatting away the unappealing butterflies. Do this for one or two minutes, holding and swatting the butterflies.
- Notice any thoughts and sensations in your body as you hold one hand open and swat with the other hand.

Imagine trying to continue holding one hand open and allowing butterflies to gently land in your palm while swatting other butterflies away at the same time. Could you continue doing this for a long time?

Would you be able to live your life? It may be difficult to do the things you do as you struggle to hold onto things and at the same time push things away. Thoughts can be like the butterflies. If you try to hold them for too long or attempt to push them away, they will overwhelm you. However, if you are willing to begin observing thoughts and other inner sensations (regardless of how they make you feel) as if they are butterflies landing in the palm of your hand, they will eventually fly away, making room for other thoughts and experiences to present themselves. Move onto the next exercise as you continue your metamorphosis.

Unfolding Your Wings

- Sit comfortably at the front edge of a chair and close your eyes. Bring your awareness to the natural rhythm and flow of your breath as you spend a few moments inhaling and exhaling.
- Bring to mind a recent situation where you felt pain and had an urge to avoid or control it. It may have been a moment when the fear kicked in, right before an activity, and you froze or decided to flee. Visualize this situation in your mind. Where were you? Who was with you? What was happening? Notice how it feels to think about this experience. Then, notice how it feels to experience the present moment as you sit in your chair.
- Now, in your mind, return to the situation that caused pain and notice any fear or anxiety that comes up. Notice any changes in your body, including tension, tightness, tingling, pain, a knot in your stomach, or any other physical sensation. What is your mind telling you about these sensations? There may be many different sensations occurring at the same time. Allow them to be present and notice if you begin to judge them as good or bad, harmful or unwanted.
- Next, bring your awareness to your urge to act on the sensations. Notice if you want to wiggle or change positions. Notice if you want the experience to stop or if you have an urge to flee or retreat. Notice if parts of your body (maybe even your whole body) are becoming tense, tight, closed and restricted. Where is the tension and tightness located?
- Now, stepping into vulnerability, begin to slowly but steadily open up and allow any unpleasant sensation in. Sit up straight, lift your chin and widen across your chest a little. Next, lift your arms out to the sides, opening them wide. Breathe deep, opening up to the full experience without trying to fight or control or get rid of any unpleasant sensations. Stay here for a few moments, arms wide open, chest and chin lifted, breathing deeply and bringing patience, kindness and compassion to the experience, as you would do for a child or a friend who was in pain.
- Notice as the feeling of struggle and restriction ebbs and flows.
- Notice as the feeling of ease and openness ebbs and flows as well.

The purpose of this exercise is to teach you that pain and fear come and go. Persistent pain, or any sustained unpleasant physical or emotional experience, can cause us to withdraw and isolate from life. It can feel like the butterfly in its cocoon. It may feel safe, but how long have you been stuck and what purpose has the cocoon served? How has the cocoon affected your relationships, health, work and life?

Are you ready to spread your wings and set out to explore life? Change is not always easy, but the pain and difficulty that it takes to grow will pass. What is one small action you can take today to emerge from the cocoon and begin to experience and enjoy the freedom of living the life you deserve? Commit to opening up to the struggle. Notice the urge to retreat to the safety of your cocoon. Notice the urge to rush to break through the cocoon. Completing this exercise is an act of courage. If you spread your wings and do something new and somewhat difficult, you will find renewed confidence and resilience in your abilities, and gain a wider experience of life.

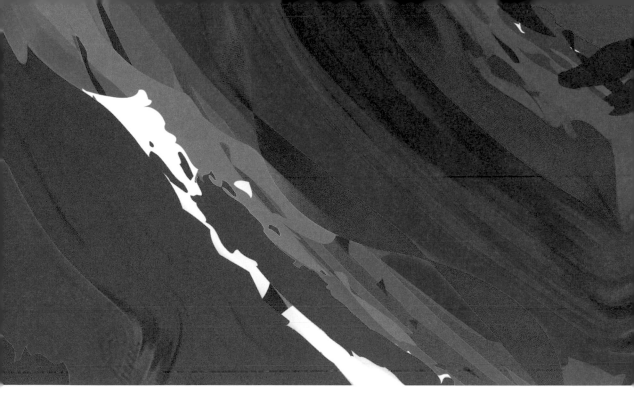

PART IV

Fully Present and Aware:
Be in the Moment and Relate Differently

"It's like you're surfing... The same wave that can be a source of pain
can be a beautiful flowing grace and source of power.
It's all a matter of how you respond to it."
— Trey Anastasio

CHAPTER 20: AWAKENING THE BODY

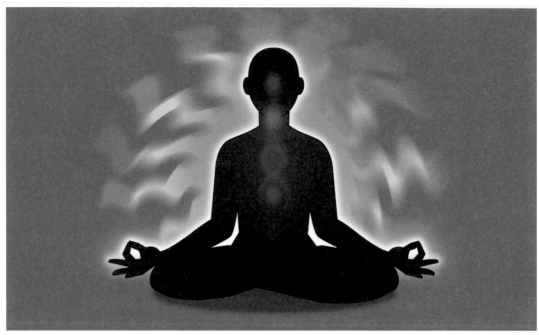

You can learn to notice all sensations in the body with curiosity and kindness.

Many of us have become accustomed to numbing our pain and other unwanted sensations because that is what we've been conditioned to do. We might have grown up watching parents, caregivers and role models distract or attempt to suppress pain by numbing themselves to it. They may have struggled to cope with the challenges in their lives and may even have used addictive substances or behaviors to numb out their feelings.

Many of our habits are learned by witnessing the behavior of others. When we watch these patterns play out over and over again, we eventually may pick up certain habits that we repeat in our own lives. We often don't question our patterns because they've become second nature for us. We've been programmed to follow them, and we default to them instinctively assuming it's the best way to handle things. We become so familiar with these patterns that we might never even consider doing things differently.

Avoidance of uncomfortable bodily sensations is common for those living with pain. The desire to eliminate pain can lead people to seek magic bullet solutions including drugs, alcohol, isolation, obsessive thoughts and so on. When these "cures" don't work, anxiety and uncertainty increase and so does the bodily discomfort. The Protector Within might even lobby for being "right," continually placing pain control at the top of the goal list. However, goals that involve never again feeling something: "I don't want to feel bad anymore," or, "I don't want to worry anymore," are called "Dead Men's Goals" because only a dead man is capable of achieving them.

The next practice involves exploring physical sensations by opening up to what your mind and body offer. These sensations may be pleasant, unpleasant or neutral. The aim is to stay present with whatever sensation arises whether it's a feeling of lightness, heaviness, numbness, tingling, burning in your chest or butterflies in your stomach. Simply be with any desire to resist or struggle in your body and mind.

As you practice this exercise, remember that you are learning to live life with all sensations, pleasant or unpleasant, painful or not. Notice all sensations with curiosity and kindness. Opening yourself up to feeling these sensations is one of the most important steps you can take as it can help you transform your relationship with whatever bodily sensations arise.

 ## Observing Bodily Sensations

- Wearing comfortable, loose clothing, find a quiet place to sit where you won't be disturbed. You may decide to do a few stretches to prepare the body for stillness. Sit on a cushion or chair and move forward on the seat with your spine straight, but not too stiff. Approach this exercise with a sense of curiosity and a readiness to explore the sensations of this amazing body of yours, noticing the energy that it brings into each moment. You can explore different levels of sensation in the body scan: the surface level, where you might feel the air temperature and pressure, moving down to the level of the muscles. You might even feel to the level of bone. As you scan throughout the body, you may find that there are places where you feel no sensation at all. Just notice and be present.

Now, let's begin the body scan.

- Close your eyes and take a deep breath in and then exhale. Bring your awareness to the very top of your head. See if you can get a felt sense of the triangular section from the forehead back to the back of the skull, where a crown would gently rest. As you focus your awareness on that part of the skull, see if you notice any sensations. You may feel air, pressure, a slight buzzy feeling, or a feeling of energy in the area. Or, you might feel nothing at all.

- Next, bring your awareness to the right side of your head, including your right ear. Focus on that section of the skull for a few moments. Some of us have pushed away sensation in the body, so it may take some time to re-sensitize ourselves, to feel what is present. We may not even be aware that we are feeling a particular sensation until we compare one place with another.

- Then, slowly move your awareness to the left side of your head, including your left ear. Notice if there's any difference between the two sides. Remember that nothing needs to change; simply notice.

- Move now to the back of the skull and down to the neck. This is an area we don't pay much attention to. See if you can get a felt sense of that area. What sensations are present?

- Now, let's experience sensations in the face, an area where we're more used to feeling sensation. First, notice the left and right sides of your forehead. Can you feel the energy that makes up that part of your face? Move your attention down to your eyes. Open and close your eyelids focusing on how they feel. Can you feel your eyeballs and maybe even gain a felt sense of the sockets of the eyes, deep in your head?

- Move to your cheeks. Are they relaxed or tense? You might feel the sinus cavities deep behind the cheekbones. Now move to your nose. Can you feel the very tip of your nose? How about the rest of it? As you move down your face, notice your jaw. You might separate the teeth ever so slightly, and very gently move the jaw side to side and notice: Is it loose? Is it tight? What are you feeling in that area? Bring your awareness to your mouth. Without moving them, can you feel your lips? How about your teeth entering your gums? The hard and soft palates? Notice where your tongue is in your mouth. Is it relaxed at the bottom of your mouth, or is it pressed tightly to the roof? The tongue is one of the hardest working muscles in the body and it's a very good indicator of how much tension you are holding. Now, for a moment gently press your tongue to the roof of your mouth and notice if you feel your entire body tensing. Now relax your tongue at the bottom of your mouth.
- As you move through the body scan, return to the tongue now and again, simply noticing: Is it still relaxed at the bottom of your mouth, or has it tensed? Just notice.
- Now move to the large muscles in the neck that hold up your head. Notice what you are feeling there. Start by scanning the front of the neck, then around to the right side, to the back and finally return your awareness to the front. Can you get a felt sense of the energy in that area of the body?
- Move now to the shoulders and simply notice: are they relaxed, or are they inching up toward your ears? Nothing needs to change. Just notice and feel what is present.
- Now, check in with both arms, comparing one side to the other. Focus on the upper arms, where your arms connect with your shoulders. Move down to the elbows and the lower arms.
- Now check in with the wrists and the hands; we'll work through the hands in sections. Notice the backs of your hands. You might feel pressure where your hands are resting on your knees. Notice what else is present. Now, notice the palms of your hands. Can you feel the energy of life in your palms? Finally, without moving them, can you get a felt sense of each of your fingers? How about your index fingers? Your middle fingers? Your ring fingers? And your pinkies? Your thumbs? Stop for a moment and feel the energy in the hands and up the arms.
- Now move to the front of the torso. Notice any feelings in the chest. Move down and see if you can get a felt sense of the midriff, the area just above the waist. What about the abdominal area—are you holding the belly tight, or is it loose and relaxed? Just notice.
- Notice where the breath is in the body. Is it deep in the belly or abdominal area? Is it higher in the chest? Is it someplace in-between? Simply notice.
- Return to the shoulders and move down the back of the body. Bring your awareness to the upper back, an area where the body sometimes holds tension. Notice what is present in this moment. Move to the midback, the area above the waist. What about the lower back, below the waist? Now notice the buttocks. Feel the sits bones pressing into your cushion or your chair. Notice the area of the groin or saddle and the perineum.

- Now move both your legs and compare one side with the other. Bring your awareness to the thighs. Scan each side and notice any differences or sensations, including the pressure of the cushion or chair you're sitting on. Do you feel the energy in that section of the body? Just notice.
- Check in with your knees, calves and shins.
- Now move back to the upper part of the torso again, front and back, left and right. What sensations do you feel there? Have the sensations changed since you scanned them earlier? Simply be present and notice.
- Notice your ankles and feet. First, bring your awareness to the tops of your feet. You may feel pressure if you are sitting with your legs crossed. Or, maybe you feel the air temperature. See if you can feel the energy behind it all. Notice the heels, the arch and the ball of each foot. Without moving them, can you feel the big toes? How about the second toes? The middle toes? The fourth toes? The little toes? Scan through your entire body and notice if there are areas where you can still feel the aliveness, and then perhaps areas where the energy has decreased.
- See if you can hold the feeling of energy throughout the whole body at one time.
- Now, for a moment, let's move inside the body. Can you sense your spine? Use your awareness to travel up and down the spine several times, sensing the strength and solidity of the spine and the energy moving through it.
- Now, feel the consistent and reliable beat of your heart, faithfully pumping blood without any attention from you. Can you feel its rhythm, similar to that of your breath?
- See if you can get a felt sense of the diaphragm muscle and notice how effortless your breath is as you are being breathed.
- Now allow your awareness to move through your entire body. Take a moment and try to hold the experience of whatever is present or not present, pleasant or unpleasant. Sink into whatever sensation it is that comes up for you.

Feel free to remain in this space as long as you wish. Take a moment to acknowledge your practice. You might like to journal about what you experienced during the body scan and write about what you noticed. Be gentle with yourself as you go about your daily activities.

Practicing a body scan regularly can help you "feel into" life better by paying attention to the sensations happening in your body. In other words, it can help you stay with what is present, even if your mind tells you that it doesn't "feel" like it. We open to difficult or unpleasant sensations in service of our values. Can you allow sensations to be as they are and observe them curiously while you do what's important? This can open up possibilities for moving your body in new ways, decreasing fear about your body, and allowing you to be more active as you explore the world. This exercise can also teach you to feel the sensations your body is offering and to be with those sensations, accepting them and allowing the process to unfold. The more you practice, the easier it becomes to actively listen to the body and mind and notice uncomfortable, comfortable and neutral sensations. Instead of ignoring or distracting from sensations of pain or discomfort this can help you build trust that it's safe to experience all types of feelings in your body.

CHAPTER 21: RIDE THE WAVE

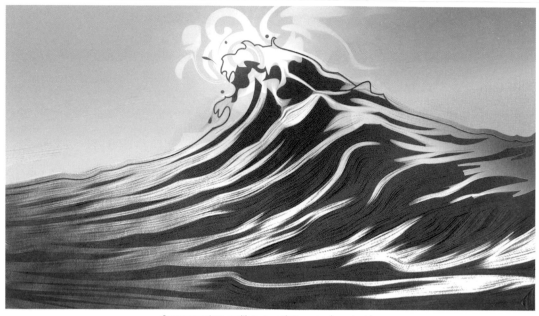

Strong emotions are like waves that you can learn to ride.

People living with pain often have strong emotions. Pain is an emotional experience and unpleasant emotions are part of pain. Half of all people with pain also struggle with anxiety and depression and many people are overly medicated in an attempt to ease unpleasant emotions. Even narcotic opioids, which are prescribed for physical pain, are now being prescribed for emotional pain—which many people in the medical community feel is unacceptable. Two thirds of the normal human emotions we experience do not feel good. Feelings like fear, anger, anxiety, sadness, guilt and disgust are not pleasant. There exists a gap between the emotions we often experience and what we are willing to have. It's not as if we have an internal keyboard of emojis and if a strong emotion arises we can just delete it and choose the next smiley face.

Facing unpleasant emotions and returning to life can be like swimming in the ocean. You head to the water with plenty of advice running through your mind: "Don't forget the sunscreen." "Stay between the buoys." "Don't swim for 30 minutes after eating." "Watch out for sharks!" You know what to do and you launch headlong into the water expecting to have a fun and relaxing time. As you dive in head-first and splash around, your fun is suddenly interrupted by strong feelings of fear and anxiety, causing you to panic. It feels as if you've been knocked off your feet by the undertow and you can no longer touch the sandy bottom.

As you are being pulled out into the deep dark ocean your mind sets the goal, "I must get back to shore." Without thinking, your instincts kick in and you take immediate action. You start paddling furiously against the rip. As soon as it seems you are making a little progress you start to tire and realize you are losing the battle. You swim harder, roll over on your back and kick with your legs, but you are getting nowhere fast. As you struggle to get back to shore, you forget why you came to the beach in the first place.

Negative thoughts fill your head: "If only I had stayed between the buoys." "I should have practiced swimming before coming to the beach." "What a risky mistake I've made." Wondering how you got here and thinking about what you should have done differently is no help. You continue paddling furiously but get nowhere. You call for help hoping the lifeguard will come to the rescue.

Does pain make you feel like you're struggling against the current in the ocean? My job is not to rescue you, but to teach you to rescue yourself. The thing about pain is that you can get sucked into a riptide at any time. That rip may be depression, anxiety, the urge to overeat,

fear of activity, physical pain, or the use of drugs to numb yourself. I want you to learn how to get out of trouble when you get stuck in an emotional rip.

I invite you to swim slowly across the rip. I promise to swim alongside you. As you do this you will feel the tug of the rip. You will get carried out to sea further than you'd like and your mind will flash all sorts of scary scenarios before your eyes. That's what minds do. Mine does it too. I'm not asking you not to be scared or anxious. I'm asking you to swim across the rip while experiencing those thoughts and emotions. Put on your mental wet suit and give the next exercise a try.

 ## Surfing Emotions

Emotions always come in waves. Sometimes they come in a small ripple and other times they roll in like a powerful tsunami that knocks you off your feet. Emotion-surfing can help you learn to willingly be with the difficult and unpleasant emotions and their triggers. These waves are usually short-lived and by learning to surf and ride these emotions it can help you stop engaging in activities that make emotions worse like emotion suppression, ruminating, and engaging in emotion-driven behavior.

Sit comfortably in a chair or on a cushion. Close your eyes if it feels comfortable and try this activity to help you connect with an unpleasant bodily sensation.

- See if you can connect to an unpleasant bodily sensation. Notice where it is and notice where it is most intense. Just simply notice and breathe into it.
- Can you describe the sensation?
- What are the emotions that go with that sensation?
- Notice where this feeling is in your body and see if you can open yourself up to it a little. Give the feeling some space. Breathe with the feeling.
- Chances are you do not like this feeling but try to let it be for a moment. You don't have to like it—just allow it to be present for a few moments. You may want to place your hand on it.
- Notice if the feeling shrinks or disappears. If this happens that is fine, but it is not the goal. The aim of the exercise is simply to be with whatever feeling is present.
- Notice if the feeling gets bigger or stronger. No matter how intense or big the feeling seems, it can't get bigger than you. Breathe into it and make more room for it with each breath.
- Where are you on the wave? How strong is the emotion?
- If this feeling were an object what would it look like?
- Do you have any urges? What does the feeling make you want to do? See what it's like to notice the urge without acting on it.

Be aware that despite your best efforts, you can still get stuck in a rip. Tides may change, or maybe a huge wave comes and knocks you off your feet. Once you're in a rip you have an important choice to make: Keep struggling and eventually succumb to exhaustion and the possibility of drowning or stop struggling and take effective action by swimming across the rip towards your values.

It is normal and natural to have painful feelings and emotions; we all have them. The practice of emotion-surfing helps you observe and willingly approach all parts of your emotional experience. Instead of reacting to unpleasant emotions, or trying to control or change them, you can learn to lean into the pain.

Emotion-surfing promotes mindful awareness and an ability to observe and accept all parts of the emotion: sensations, thoughts, feelings and urges. Eventually, you will find your way to calm water and be able to enjoy life again. This lesson in emotion-surfing is an invitation to give up paddling furiously and willingly ride the emotions and scary thoughts that often come with pain.

This is an invitation to reconnect with what really matters—the people and activities in life that you enjoy. It is an invitation to surf and take effective action based on the situation you are in at any given moment. If you're feeling safe and happy, it means enjoying the sun and surf. If you're stuck in a riptide of difficult emotions, it means letting go of the struggle and taking small strokes in the direction of your goals, simply being with whatever experiences come up. There may be one big wave or many smaller ones. Leaning into the wave will prevent it from knocking you over.

CHAPTER 22: CULTIVATING COMPASSION

Pain can start at a very young age and chronic pain in children and adolescents is on the rise. Children who consume too much sugar and junk food, spend too much time in front of screens, and don't get enough physical activity are prone to a host of chronic conditions. Obesity and diabetes can begin at a young age and can contribute to pain in adulthood. Childhood arthritis, back pain, and poor physical development are real. Yet, the reasons why our little ones hurt can run much deeper. Long-lasting neglect, social disadvantage, and severe economic hardship creates an environment of toxic stress; children in specific racial or ethnic groups are disproportionately affected.

Other experiences that can weigh heavily on our kids include living with violence in the home, bullying (both online and offline), discrimination, poverty and community violence. Living with a family member who is mentally ill or who abuses alcohol or drugs can be traumatizing for children. Certain childhood events are especially likely to cause trauma, including the sudden loss of a family member, a natural disaster, or a violent event such as a school shooting. Studies show that such experiences can have serious consequences, especially when they occur early in life or when a series of these events happen over time. However, these types of events do not predestine children to poor health, and most children are able to recover when they have the right support—particularly the presence of a warm, sensitive caregiver.

After a traumatic event, a child may experience strong negative emotions like fear or helplessness, and physiological symptoms like anxiety, headaches and stomachaches may develop soon afterward and continue well beyond the initial event. Childhood trauma has the ability to cut deep, forming an emotional wound that leaves behind a constant reminder of the need to protect themselves. When the response to trauma remains activated without the calming influence of a supportive adult, it short circuits crucial connections in the developing brain. Disrupting sensitive periods of development can lead to lifelong physical and mental health problems.

Toxic stress and trauma hurt children during a critical time when they crave affection, recognition, and validation yet feel overwhelmingly vulnerable, abandoned and unloved. Being raised in an environment where pain and suffering are persistent can sensitize the nervous system of every member of the family. Many adults with pain were raised by caregivers who also had pain. We are learning how pain may be passed down from generation to generation.

Experiencing trauma at a young age can leave a person disconnected from emotions and bodily sensations and leave them yearning for self-love and self-care. The child inside of you—tender and innocent—craves connection, safety, recognition, acceptance and unconditional love. The next exercise can be quite powerful and can help you rekindle the compassion, kindness and love you deserve.

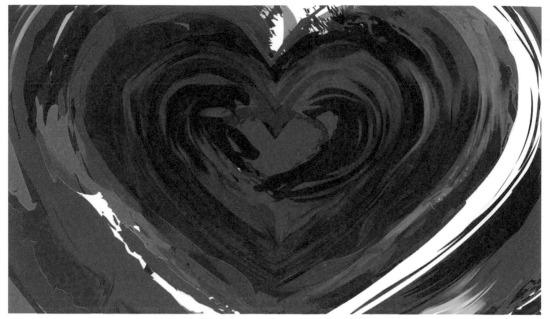

You can learn to show yourself compassion, love and kindness.

 ## Childlike Kindness

This is a longer exercise and is best performed with your eyes closed. Sit comfortably with your back straight. Close your eyes and take a few moments to focus on your breath.

- Imagine that you're going to invite someone into your space who you have had a special relationship with. It could be someone from your childhood or later in life, as long as it's someone who had caring eyes and a gentle tone of voice that communicated tender love and acceptance. Someone who had space for you in all your complexity. Identify this person and invite them into your space.

- Imagine that this person is now holding you in an unconditional way. As challenging as it may be, your job is to open up to the love and acceptance that this person offers. See if you can breathe in and open up to the feeling, sensation and knowledge that you are exactly as you should be. Nothing needs to change or be achieved at this moment and there is no one you need to impress. You are perfect exactly as you are. Breathe in and see if you can allow that feeling of acceptance to fill your whole body. Open up and allow yourself to feel accepted just as you are.

- Notice any thoughts that might be telling you you're not acceptable, or giving you lists of things to do in order to be acceptable. See if you can gather those thoughts and take them into this space of acceptance. You might also feel parts of your body tense up if negative memories or thoughts show up. See if you can open your body up, even those spaces that are tense.

- Now, visualize yourself as a child (or maybe when you first felt pain). Visualize yourself during a time when you did not feel loved and accepted. Was there a time when you were young and were not invited into a group or when you made an innocent childhood mistake? Maybe someone who you cared about said something critical. Visualize yourself at that age and let the image in your head become clear.

- Notice as you sit here now as an adult, that you have infinitely more knowledge and experience than you had as a young child.
- With the distinction between you now as the older and wiser one with all your knowledge and experience, go and visit the younger you, feeling inadequacy or pain. Imagine you're sitting next to this younger you.
- Now, with all your knowledge and experience as an adult, I'd like you to take three perspectives on what is happening.
- The first perspective will use your five senses to take in all sensations. Now, the younger you is not doing this. The younger you, with this feeling of inadequacy, has tunnel vision. She only sees certain things and feels certain things and is not taking in the whole picture. But, I'd like you here and now (the adult you) to take in the whole picture. So, visually what do you see? What do you smell? What do you hear? Is there a physical sensation?
- The second perspective involves noticing thoughts. Take a guess at what the younger you is thinking about herself and others? If you have trouble with that, have a look at her body posture—is she standing up straight or slouching? What are her eyes doing? Is she looking directly at you, or looking away? What is she doing with her hands?
- The third perspective is emotional. I'd like you as an adult, here and now, to share the emotion of inadequacy or fear with the younger you. See if you can identify where in your body you feel inadequacy. Place your hand on that part of your body.
- Now, imagine what the younger you needed, and I'd like you to give it to her. Give the younger you the unconditional love and acceptance you needed.
- Imagine that you're holding the younger you. Feel the body of the younger you in your arms. Maybe she's a bit tense, limp or trembling. Imagine that you're holding the younger you, unconditionally and open-heartedly giving love and acceptance. Without any judgment, simply openly give. Give her what she needs as long as she needs it. There's no time-limit here; stay and give as long as it's needed. Imagine what that would feel like for you to help in this way.
- Now that you've imagined the thoughts, feelings and sensations of the younger you, I'd like you to imagine embodying the younger you. It's not easy, not much room there. But in this impulsive body filled with reactivity you can help her now. You are going to do a special thing to help her. I'd like you to imagine, take a deep breath, and help her break out of that locked position she has been in. So, breathe in as if you were a spring flower breaking through the ice and snow of a winter day, towards the sunshine. See if you can help her break loose. Take a deep breath again and help her to show her vulnerability, just like a spring flower shows its vulnerability on that early winter day. And when you help her show vulnerability, you can see all other human beings with the same vulnerability. You are not alone.

The next time you have feelings of inadequacy, see if it's possible for you to stop, breathe, put your hand on the area where you feel the inadequacy, and give yourself what you need. You don't have to wait for other people to be kind to you. You can choose to respond to your own needs anytime, anywhere by showing yourself compassion, love and kindness. Knowing that we can be loved exactly as we are gives us all the best opportunity for growing into the healthiest of people. Learning to shower yourself with compassion and kindness helps to train inner strength and build the outer life you desire.

CHAPTER 23: LETTING GO

The root of the word "forgive" comes from the Latin word "perdonare," meaning "to give completely, without reservation." Studies show that anger and resentment towards oneself, health care providers and persons blamed for accidents or trauma are part of our pain experience. In recent years, the role of anger, resentment and animosity in the persistence of pain has received growing attention.

Left unchecked, anger and resentment can lead to self-destructive behavior, such as heavy drinking, painful isolation, self-harm such as cutting oneself, or acts of hatred. Sometimes the self-blame is simply about not living the life we would like to live. It keeps us stuck.

The act of forgiveness is a common element of spiritual teachings. Although forgiveness is a particularly challenging and sensitive topic, especially for trauma survivors, it can be healing medicine for those who suffer. Most people think of forgiveness as a feeling that comes along with telling someone that you forgive them for a transgression or harmful act. However, seen through the lens of ACT, forgiveness is not a feeling. Forgiveness means to "give what went before the harm." In this sense, forgiveness is an action, not a feeling.

Spiritual leader Marianne Williamson begins each day by asking herself in her morning prayer who she needs to forgive. She teaches that we can hold a grievance, or pursue peace of mind, but it is difficult to do both. When we hold onto our grievances, replaying the same story about our misfortunes, it pulls us back in time. It keeps us from defusing from fearful thoughts and feelings of hatred, revenge or injustice.

Each time we re-embody the past, it drives the second arrow in deeper. The first arrow is the initial, physical pain we experience, but this second arrow is our suffering and represents our reaction. The suffering can bring on feelings of rage, hurt, panic and fear. Physical sensation takes hold of the body—muscles clench, cheeks flush, temperature skyrockets, the stomach turns, and the mind goes into overdrive. When you experience these intense sensations, you may become deaf to anything anyone is saying, only hearing your own narrative racing through your mind. Shame, self-blame, guilt, regret and remorse rein free. The only person who suffers when you are unable to surrender to forgiveness is you, and the longer your heart stays closed, the more difficult it is to take action.

Forgiveness is not about condoning, excusing, or even forgetting. Forgiveness is a choice you can make to abandon resentment and offer benevolence in the face of unfairness. It's likely you won't forget the event but if you can forgive, you may remember the event in new ways—without continuing to harbor deeply held anger and other negative emotions.

Forgiveness can shift negative emotions to positive ones and can provide a sense of relief, lightness, peace and ease. Feelings of calm and joy are welcomed, while negative emotions like anger, anxiety and sadness decrease. This doesn't mean the negative feelings around the event will be gone forever—these feelings may come and go. Forgiveness is a process, an act you can choose to take in order to help yourself feel lighter and happier. Your forgiveness doesn't have to be about the other person, it's something you do for you.

Five Steps Toward Forgiveness

Sit comfortably with your feet flat on the floor and rest your hands on your legs with your palms facing up. Close your eyes if that feels comfortable, otherwise gently look down about a foot or two in front of you.

Step 1: Anchor to the Present Moment

Spend a moment taking some slow, steady, deep breaths in and out. As you're breathing, allow your shoulders, hands, legs and feet to relax. Allow your body to feel heavy, sinking into your seat. Take a moment to connect with your breath moving in and out as your belly rises and falls. During this exercise I'll ask some questions; at any time, you can return to the safety and anchor of your breath.

Step 2: Pause to Reflect

Take a few moments to reflect on the following questions and pause for several seconds after you've answered each question: Where is there tension in my life? What am I holding a grudge about? Who am I holding a grudge against? When in life do I feel I was wronged? Choose just one past event or person that leaves you feeling angry or resentful.

Step 3: Observe Without Judgement

Stay with the event or person who has caused you to feel angry or resentful and continue breathing deeply. As you are breathing, notice and name one thought you're experiencing. (Pause 5 seconds). Next, notice and name one bodily sensation you are experiencing. (Pause 5 seconds). Notice and name one emotion. (Pause 5 seconds). Finally, step outside this experience and take the observer perspective. Find that safe place where you can notice your thoughts and feelings as you watch this entire experience.

Step 4: Develop a New Perspective

Who has the power to let go of the grievance you hold? Who is getting hurt by holding on? What have you given up because you are stuck in this struggle? If you were to give yourself the life that was possible before the distressing event, what would that life look like? What actions would you take toward yourself and those who are important to you?

Step 5: Actively Affirm

Place both hands on your heart and repeat this statement silently to yourself, or you can say it out loud: "I will work to forgive those who have harmed me. If I've harmed anyone, knowingly or unknowingly, I ask their forgiveness." As you repeat this phrase, notice the feelings, thoughts or bodily sensations that come up. Don't analyze them, don't judge them, simply allow your feelings to be.

Bring your awareness back to your breath for a moment and then bring in the second phrase. You can say this silently to yourself or you can say it out loud: "If anyone has hurt or harmed me, knowingly or unknowingly, I forgive them." Gently turn toward any feeling, image or memory that bubbles to the surface and allow it to be in the space with you as you observe.

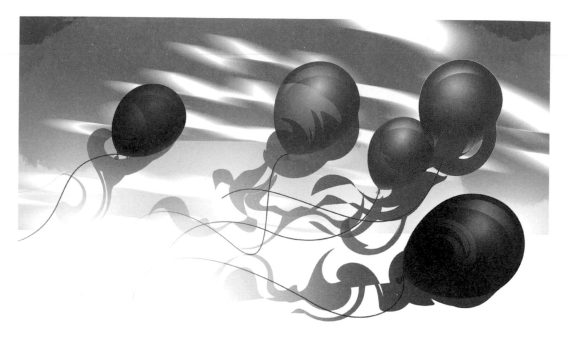

Forgiveness is an act of letting go and can make you feel lighter and happier.

Finally, turn your attention to forgiveness of yourself. You may be wrapped up in self-blame or perfectionism. Repeat this statement silently to yourself or you can say it out loud: "For all the ways that I have hurt or harmed myself, knowingly or unknowingly, I offer myself forgiveness."

Spend about 60 seconds in silence, breathing deeply. Take a nice, deep breath in and bring your awareness to your belly, noticing how it rises and falls as you breathe. Allow the feelings that this experience brings to come and go. Wiggle your fingers and toes to start bringing activity back into your body. Roll your shoulders back, and when you're ready, open your eyes.

You may have noticed your breathing or pulse quicken during certain parts of the exercise. This may be an indication of an area that requires more exploration. What painful thoughts, judgments, feelings or memories do you have to let go of? Forgiveness is not a single action. It is a series of acts freely chosen by the forgiver. Forgiveness is a gradual process that does not need to involve the offender. It is done to release yourself from the struggle with negative thoughts and feelings to help you feel lighter, happier and better able to move forward with your life.

CHAPTER 24: BEND THE RULES

People living with pain are often dissatisfied with the care, information and treatment they receive from the medical system. It can take upwards of five years and seeing more than 10 practitioners before someone with pain finds a safe, acceptable and useful treatment. It may be even more challenging to find a practitioner who is empathetic and who you can create a lasting relationship with. How many practitioners have you seen for the care of your pain? Five years and 10 practitioners is too many, and chances are you have received different diagnoses, opposing opinions, and ritualistic rules as to what you should and should not do for your pain. This can keep you stuck in the analysis paralysis mode, unsure as to the cause of your pain, unsure where to turn for help and unable to take action and move forward with your life.

In earlier chapters, you learned that the mind is a problem-solving machine; always taking in information, evaluating problems, and broadcasting ways to solve them. Another critical function of the problem-solving mind is rule making. Humans rely heavily on our interactions with others—and with our environment—to avoid chaos, harm and pain and to thrive and survive in the world. In these interactions, the human mind creates rules to establish appropriate and acceptable ways to act and respond.

For example, when waiting in line, we follow the rule of "one person at a time," and expect others to do the same. We get upset if someone cuts in line because they have violated a rule. These rules create a measurable amount of safety for us, and the mind loves safety. As a general rule, it's safer to drive under the speed limit versus speeding, to avoid walking where a "wet floor" sign is to prevent a fall, and to take your medicine as prescribed. The mind is excellent at following rules.

Yet, when the protective thinking mind dictates how we should act it sometimes creates rules that don't serve us. Based on your own life experience with pain, as well as the opinions of others, you've probably created some rules around pain. If you need a reminder, turn back to Chapter 16, where we covered thoughts and what your thoughts lead to.

In short, rules are made to be broken, or at least bent a little as you test the waters. If we follow the mind's rules about pain and stay within the bounds of these rules, new horizons might never be explored. Say for example, you are someone who lives with chronic lower back pain and have been told that the lower back is a delicate part of the body, you should never bend your back and always bend from the waist. Imbedded within this thinking may be the rule of "never bend the back, always bend from the waist." This rule is based on a very outdated mechanical view of the joints in the lower spine being weak and unstable and that it is safer to bend with the hips (practitioner opinions may have even contributed to the formation of this rule). This rule is false, and science tells us the spine is designed to move, flex, and bend and that the structure of the human spine was designed for lifelong resilience.

As a consequence of believing this rule, you may fear basic daily activities like tying your shoes, cleaning and certain types of exercise. Your mind might whisper in your ear or yell at you, "don't bend over" or, "only bend from the waist." It might also tell you not to join that gentle yoga class because the instructor said you would be doing exercises that make the back more flexible. These rules go beyond the physical. You may have created a rule that you will not apply for a job because you have a physical challenge, and you think that no one wants to hire someone with a disability. The idea that you are unworthy of gainful employment, or that no one will value your contribution and skills, prevents you from working and advancing your career.

When you realize how these thoughts and rules about pain impact your life, you begin to judge them differently. When you realize that a thought such as "no one wants to hire someone with pain" is causing a lot of stress, you can begin to counter it with "I am worthy of employment." These statements may seem unreasonable and illogical based on how the mind works. However, as you begin to break or bend the rules, you will begin to see how the mind can unintentionally contribute to your suffering.

The outcomes of following these rules are apparent in our language and often show up as objections and reasons as to why we can't do something. You can become more aware of this in your thoughts or speech by noticing the word "but." It seems like such a small, insignificant word. It's only three letters. What harm can it do? Using the word "but" in the middle of a sentence can negate everything that came before it. The next exercise will show you how to create powerhouse statements that help bend the rules, will kick your inner critic, calm the Protector Within and help you to behave in a way that is in line with your goals and dreams.

 Kick Your Buts

In this exercise you will learn how to kick some "buts." We use the word "but" because in some way it runs counter to our rule-making minds. For example, you might say "I would like to go to the Tai Chi class at the gym, but I am in so much pain." In the statement above, the word "but" indicates there is no way for you to attend the Tai Chi class because of your pain. Use the lines provided below to write down your "but" thoughts about things you would like to do *but* you avoid because your mind has inserted a rule and is holding you back.

If you are having a hard time finding any "but" statements look back to Chapter 15 . Track your thoughts and "but" statements over the next week and see if you can fill in 5-10 on the lines below.

Example: "I would like to go to dinner with my friends, but I am in so much pain."
Example: "I would like to go back to work, but I am in so much pain."

_____but _____

_____but _____

_____but _____

_____but _____

_____but _____

_____but _____

_____but _____

Now let's kick for the goalposts and replace every "but" with the word "and." Rewrite your statements from above as "and" statements.

Example: "I would like to go to dinner with my friends, and I am in so much pain."
Example: "I would like to go back to work, and I am in so much pain."

_____and _____

_____and _____

_____and _____

_____and _____

_____and _____

_____and _____

_____and _____

Paying attention to the rules your mind makes and then changing one small three-letter word is one way to overcome the influence of thoughts. Words and language can have an impact on your behavior, and becoming a mindful observer of your own thoughts, words and rules can have a dramatic impact. It alters the meaning of thoughts in a very subtle but radical way. Substituting "but" with "and" implies that you can take meaningful action in life even if you have pain. How would following this new rule instead of the one your mind has offered up as a solution impact your life? You may have noticed that in these sentences, the activities that are meaningful to you are listed first, before pain. That's because you and your life are what's important, and should always come first, before pain—another radical idea.

CHAPTER 25: BIGGER THAN PAIN

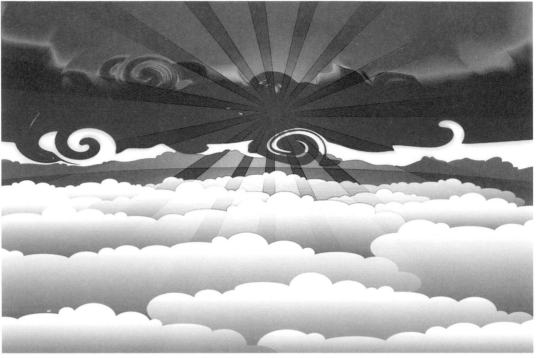

Be the observer and rise above painful thoughts, feelings and sensations.

When overwhelmed with intense or unpleasant thoughts and feelings, it can be difficult to see the distinction between you and your inner experiences. It is possible to actively notice thoughts, feelings and bodily sensations without reacting. This is one of the benefits of mindfulness practice. Without the cultivation of this skill, our inner struggles seem very close, and we become one with them. It is like two red hot pieces of fused metal. It is difficult to see where one piece begins and the other ends. Instead of having thoughts, feelings and sensations we become fused with our thoughts, feelings and sensations. This keeps us trapped, thinking we are our thoughts and feelings and can lead us into more suffering.

Practicing mindfulness helps you become more skilled at being an outside observer of your thoughts, feelings and sensations as they come and go. Similar to migrating birds or clouds floating by, thoughts have their own pattern. Just like birds and the sky, you notice thoughts and feelings from a distance. If you are noticing thoughts and feelings, and the space between you and your experience, then there must be a distinction between you and them. You have thoughts and feelings, but they are not you. Likewise, pain is not you. You may have pain, but it is not you.

Developing this observer perspective reveals you are the container for thoughts and feelings but you are not thoughts or feelings themselves. This can help you see all the different changing contexts of your life and locate a stable unchanging part of you. This part of you is constant no matter how beautiful or turbulent your inner or outer world becomes.

Like clouds in the sky, thoughts, feelings and bodily sensations come and go on their own. You can't control them. You can't change them, and you can't make them go away. But you can learn to observe them without judgment and without becoming them. The next exercise will help you develop this observer perspective and locate a stable, unchanging part of yourself. By learning how to step into the observer's shoes, you can create a non-threatening place that is safe from harm to help you approach life in the moment, with or without pain.

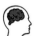

Sky and the Weather

Let's imagine that the struggle with your thoughts and feelings is like the sky and the weather. The weather is constantly changing. Some days the clouds are white and puffy and gently float through the sky. Other days they are dark and stormy. You are like the sky; you are infinite and expansive. You can watch the weather and contain it all. The white fluffy clouds, the dark and stormy clouds and everything in between. There is a part of you that can watch it all, and no matter how the weather changes, the sky will always be there, untouched by the turbulent weather.

Your observer self is like the sky, and your thoughts and feelings are like the weather. The weather changes continually, but no matter how bad it gets, the weather cannot harm the sky. If we rise high enough above the clouds–even the thickest, darkest thunderclouds–sooner or later we will reach clear sky, stretching in all directions, boundless and pure. This is a safe place, no matter how stormy the weather becomes, it cannot harm you. You are bigger than pain, bigger than thoughts or emotions and bigger than all the sensations you experience. And you may be the most important part because, without the sky, there is no weather.

More and more, you can learn to access this part of you, a safe space from which to observe and make room for difficult thoughts, feelings and sensations. A place that is safe from harm and will always be there. Pain is not all of you. When you find yourself caught up in the thunderclouds and are flooded with scary and difficult sensations, step back as you might step back and look at clouds, passing traffic or a leaf floating down a stream. Look at these sensations from the safe sanctuary of your observer self. From there, you have room and can make space for it all, even the most difficult thoughts, feelings, memories or sensations. As you practice stepping back and defusing you ultimately realize they can no longer hurt you. From here you can make choices that come from all of you and move in directions that give you vitality. Therein lies freedom from pain.

Living with chronic pain can prevent you from embracing life fully or cause you to sweep future plans under the rug. What have you put on hold because of the thought of facing pain is too much to bear? Giving up and resigning to the notion that you can't do anything about pain can make your life feel like a form of passive submission. Kneeling to raise the white flag of surrender in hopes of negotiating with pain or seeing it fully retreat rarely works. Refusing to acknowledge pain, look at pain, or accept its presence in your life may make it advance even closer. In many ways, throwing in the towel signals that you gave in to the struggle. It is like you are turning your head, torso, legs and entire body away from pain. By now you know this pivot away from pain is futile.

A willingness approach allows you to actively face pain, look at it directly and learn to take a new perspective. When you turn toward pain to face it and take a close look, you begin to see it is much more than just a single sensation; you begin to see all the different colors and layers.

Facing and embracing pain isn't easy, but with some practice, you can see it for what it is and not what it says it is. You may even begin to see that you contain these layers but aren't defined by them, and even though pain is part of your experience, it isn't your only experience. Facing the pain monster and becoming curious is one way to end the tug-of-war. The first move is to step back and get into the observer seat. Each of us has created our own unique big-and-ugly pain monster. This exercise will teach you to face pain when it rears its ugly head and is a way to look at it from a distance and see it for what it is.

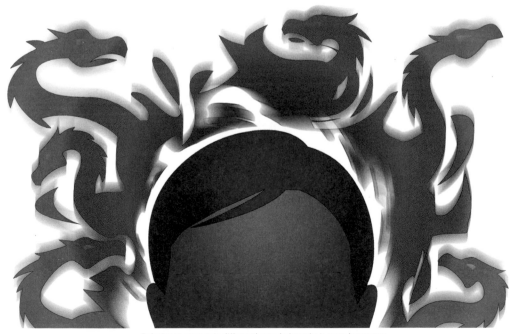

Relating to your pain differently can help make it seem less scary.

Creating Your Pain Monster

- Find a comfortable seated position with your feet firmly on the ground and your back straight. Place your hands in your lap. Roll your shoulders back and take a nice deep breath in, gently closing your eyes.
- Now, scan your body from head to toe, and when you come to a place that's painful, I'd like you to stop for a few moments. As you pause, simply name it by saying the word "pain." Take a few moments and slowly repeat the words, "pain, pain, pain."
- As you repeat this word place some energy behind it: "Pain!"
- Now, take that sensation of pain, and in your mind's eye, see if you can pull your pain out of your body. Once it is outside of your body notice if your pain has a shape. What shape is your pain? Is it round, square or triangular? Give it any shape that comes to mind.
- Next, notice how big your pain is. If you could place it outside your body, how large would it be? Is it like a baseball, a basketball, or maybe something even bigger? Just notice.
- Now that you are visualizing the shape and size, try to visualize your pain in the shape of a monster. What color is your pain monster? Is it white? Is it red? Is it very dark? Is it changing colors?
- As you're looking at this pain monster outside of your body, notice its texture. Is it smooth? Is it sharp? Is it bumpy and lumpy? Just simply notice.
- As you're looking at this pain monster outside of your body, see if you can come in contact with its voice. If your pain monster had a voice, what would it sound like?
- Is your pain monster male or female? Young or old? Is its voice high pitched or deep? Just simply notice. As you're visualizing this pain monster outside of your body, noticing its shape and texture, how large it is, and its voice, see if it has a smell. What does your pain monster smell like?
- Finally, as your pain monster's right in front of you, outside of your body, and you're taking a really good look at it, what type of thoughts does this bring up for you? What type of feelings? What type of bodily sensations do you notice?
- If you don't like this pain monster, or even hate this pain monster, just notice that and take those feelings outside of your body, too. Notice what size, shape and color your feelings are and whether or not they have a smell, a texture or a sound. And then, see if you can—nice and easily—reach out toward your pain monster. Extend your arm, extend your hand, stay in contact with any sensation that comes up, but just reach out, one hand first and then the next, and just nice and easily place your hand around that pain monster. Start to pull it gently back toward you, gently back inside your body. And just allow your pain monster to be home with you.
- To end, scan your body from head to toe, part by part, being nice and gentle with yourself, allowing yourself to open up to any experience that you're having.

Practice this exercise one more time today. Be gentle with yourself during this exercise and know that pain is just one small part of you. Everything you just experienced is a part of you. In order to not feel pain or anger or fear you would also not have to feel happiness, joy and love. Allow any thought, feeling, or bodily sensation that arises with that notion to just be without the yearning to change it. In the presence of pain can you choose to do one thing different today that adds meaning to your life? When pain shows up again, how will you handle it differently?

CHAPTER 27: FLEXING WILLINGNESS

The work involved in overcoming pain isn't always a smooth ride. It will stir up some uncomfortable thoughts and feelings. Overcoming pain is kind of like a glass filled with mud that has settled to the bottom, and our work is to get the glass clean. How do you suppose that we could get the mud out of the glass? Scooping the mud out is probably an effective way, although the water might get murky in the process. This is similar to the scary and uncomfortable feelings that might get stirred up as you begin to make changes necessary to overcome pain. What if getting the water messy was worth it in order to get the mud out of the glass?

In Part I, we looked at how struggling against pain can make it worse. This included the pain trap of the human mind and its persistent effort to control or eliminate pain in hopes of resolving it. We also looked at common methods employed to avoid pain and how most of them are unhelpful and can sometimes even be harmful. At this point, you might be thinking, if controlling pain is not the answer and eliminating pain is not the answer, then what are the alternatives?

This chapter introduces another radical idea—letting go of the struggle with pain is the path to moving beyond it. To effectively let go of the struggle you build the willingness to be with pain and other unpleasant sensations that accompany it. Just the thought of this might be off-putting. It's kind of like inviting your least favorite relatives over for a holiday dinner. It may sound like the right thing to do but may be an action you are not ready to take. Can you choose to welcome them in, even though you don't like the fact that they came?

Before you can willingly throw open the doors and invite pain to the dinner table I want you to know that willingness to be with pain is not a switch you can flip on and off. It is not a decision your mind makes, but a skill you can learn and practice. Just as you exercise your biceps, the willingness to be with pain takes time to flex, tone and build. This is a good time to remember that how you respond to pain can forecast how severe the pain will become, along with the potential physical disability and the psychological suffering that will follow. Some have argued that your response, and how you relate to pain, is the most robust predictor of what your life will look like in the future.

Still, if you are like most people living with pain you're probably wondering, "Why would I willingly decide to be present with pain?" The Protector Within is probably starting to whisper in one ear, saying things like, "This guy wants us to learn to tolerate pain," or "Just give in to it." The Protector Within may even be starting to bargain and say things like, "Yeah, sure, I'm willing to tolerate some pain if it means the pain will go away!" What is really happening here? The Protector Within is, yet again, changing the rules and saying, "I dislike pain, so I guess I could give this approach a try."

"I suppose I can try to be more willing to feel pain, if it means I won't be in so much pain." With thoughts like this, the pain trap snaps shut right around your ankle, because if you are willing to open to pain only in order to hurt less, then you are not really willing to be with pain, and you will likely wind up hurting even more.

Yes, it sounds confusing—pain is paradoxical! If the only reason you're willing to open up and feel pain today is the hope of future pain relief tomorrow, then it won't work. Because what your willingness really means is you don't want to feel pain and you'll try all kinds of things not to have it. That's not the same as being willing to feel your pain. Another way to look at this is if you're not willing to have it, you will!

Willingness is how you actively respond to your feelings, how you actively respond to your thoughts, and how you actively respond to bodily sensations when pain arises. The goal of willingness is not to eliminate pain in order to feel better, but to open yourself up to all experiences—both pleasant and unpleasant—so that you can live your life more completely.

Willingness is just one part of the journey back to a beautiful life. You're starting to see life reappear in the distance and at the same time you notice you are standing right in the middle of a cold, muddy, smelly swamp. You say to yourself, "Gee, I didn't realize that I was going to have to walk through a swamp. It's all smelly and the mud is all mushy in my shoes. It's hard to lift my feet out of the muck and move them forward. I'm wet and cranky and tired. Why didn't anyone tell me about this swamp?" When this happens, you have a choice: abandon the journey or enter the swamp. Willingness is like that. Pain is like that and so is life. We willingly go into the swamp, not because we want to get cold and wet but because it stands between us and where we are going.

 ### Holding a Wet Cold Ice Cube

Exploring different physical sensations and the thoughts and emotions that arise from those sensations can help you find new ways to be with pain. This exercise will help you explore different sensations; you will need an ice cube to do this.

- Take a moment to find a comfortable seated position and then pick up and hold an ice cube in the palm of your hand.
- If at any point this becomes too intense, you may drop the ice cube but continue to take note of any thoughts, feelings, or sensations that you are experiencing.
- Gently close your eyes or rest your gaze on a spot on the floor in front of you. Keep the ice in the palm of your hand. This may become uncomfortable, but that's okay. Take a breath. Notice any physical sensations, thoughts, or feelings that arise, allowing them to be as they are rather than what your mind tells you they are. Simply hold them in your awareness. If you are able, explore those thoughts, feelings and physical sensations with curiosity.
- If you are experiencing discomfort, stay with the discomfort and breathe into it. If you notice yourself tensing up and resisting or pushing away from your experience, acknowledge that and try to observe whatever it is you are experiencing. Simply allow any thoughts, sensations, or feelings to exist and try to make room for them.
- Now observe and notice any physical sensations. Does your hand feel cold? Hot? How does the rest of your body feel? What other physical sensations are you experiencing?

- You may be having new thoughts along with the physical sensations. Take a minute to notice your thoughts. Are you anticipating pain or discomfort? Are you wondering how long you will be able to continue with this exercise? Are you worrying about what might happen? Are you thinking about how messy this exercise might get as the ice melts in your hand?
- As the ice melts, you may be having thoughts about how long this exercise will last and how long you'll have to hold on to this cold, wet ice cube.
- Now notice what emotions accompany your thoughts. Notice and observe any emotions you may be feeling, perhaps anxiety or fear, or maybe you're surprised. What other emotions are you experiencing?
- Take a moment to observe your breathing. Are your breaths quick and shallow, or perhaps you are taking slow, deep breaths.
- Now bring your awareness to how the ice feels. Allow yourself a moment to open up to the sensations and explore them. Notice how the sensations in your hand change ever so slightly over time. Perhaps the ice feels solid or perhaps fluid. You may notice the feeling of liquid pooling or dripping in your hand. Does the temperature change as you focus on the physical sensations in your hand?
- Are there any emotions that arise? Take note of these emotions. Don't struggle against the thoughts, the feelings or the sensations. Instead, try to open up and make room for whatever you are experiencing in this moment. Approach the sensations with curiosity. Open yourself to the physical sensations, the thoughts and the emotions that arise right now. Notice how they change over time.
- When you are ready, slowly bring your awareness back to your breath. Take a moment to be with your breath and when you are ready, put the ice cube down and take note of how you feel now.

Trying to control your most difficult thoughts and sensations is like tightly gripping an ice cube. The harder you squeeze, the messier it gets. Hold them lightly. This exercise may not yet make sense and your mind may be telling you that it doesn't apply to pain. But as you become more willing to be with all experiences and sensations you will find more opportunities to live a full life with or without pain and you will likely discover that pain becomes less of a problem.

CHAPTER 28: DISARMING THE WARRIOR

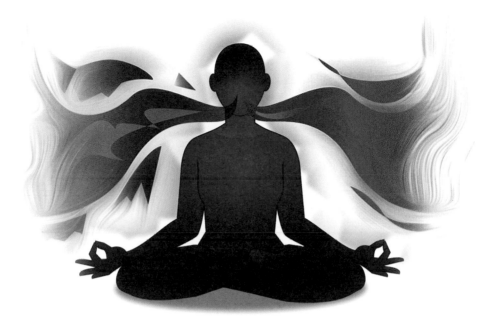

Tonglen is a meditative practice that involves taking in pain as you inhale and exhaling joy and compassion.

People living with pain are often described as fighters or warriors. Just the thought of pain is enough to put us on guard and in a defensive posture. Our response is to summon the guards to protect our sacred temple. Fortified walls go up to keep out harmful experiences, but they also serve to keep us locked in, unable to explore all that's on the other side. How does this affect our relationship with pain? You may have heard overcoming pain requires a fight. A fight for better treatment, a fight for understanding from friends and family, a fight to keep up with the demands of work or parenting, and a fight to complete everyday tasks others take for granted. Being a pain warrior drafts you into a battle that never ends.

You may not be going into a literal battle, but your mind doesn't know any different. The Protector Within dons a suit of armor and valiantly lifts her shield. No pain can penetrate this coat of steel. Unfortunately, this heavy coat of steel also blocks pleasure from getting in. Although it might make you feel safe this armor doesn't just encase your body. It also encases the soul and the heart. It's as if you've been recruited into a never-ending battle, forever stuck in the fight.

What does this look like in real life? Pain warriors have long histories of fighting pain, ignoring bodily sensations, and pushing themselves to extremes. They are more than willing to battle, stay up all night, tolerate side effects, or sit for many hours without moving. Unfortunately, practices that override the body's natural signals of discomfort can end up creating further pain. Pain warriors have survived by teaching themselves to persevere. It's how they were trained and what they were told worked. Their life of combat training probably created a compelling story driven by thoughts like, "I'm going to win this!" When our culture celebrates the fight, it reinforces the idea that this is a healthy way to handle discomfort and pain.

When pain warriors discover they have been recruited into a never-ending battle, naturally they long to handle pain differently. We work to reverse the warrior's training and surrender our shields. Taking in pain instead of pleasure and giving pleasure away instead of pain. This undoubtedly seems counterproductive. Meditation is a tool that can be used for creating this positive surrender. With practice, it wears away at our tough exterior. If living with pain is like walking around with a thick suit of armor, then meditation is the industrial-strength steel wool to rub it away. As we scour and dissolve the metal sheath around the heart it reveals our shared human vulnerability. This softens us and makes us more tender toward ourselves and others. Yes, this means we are a little raw and exposed, but there's something absolutely beautiful about connecting with life in that way. We become more aware of who we genuinely are and how we can serve others.

Tonglen

Tonglen is a meditative practice of sending and receiving. This practice involves taking in pain as you inhale and exhaling joy and compassion. During the exercise, you will work with your own pain and suffering and that of others, as well. Since it is not possible to physically inhale pain and exhale joy, this is a symbolic practice. Not only does this practice cultivate compassion, it also provides a reminder that, whether or not we see it, people deal with distress, pain and suffering every day. Thus, it helps counter our natural self-preoccupation by encouraging a shift of focus to the challenges other people face. Tonglen reverses the usual logic of avoiding pain and seeking pleasure. It is a method for overcoming our fear of suffering and for dissolving the steel around our hearts.

 Practicing with Your Own Suffering

Begin the practice with your own life. Focus on any painful situation that's real to you. It may be a current event or past hurt. You may have been angry, depressed or scared. Lean in and get caught up in the feeling as much as possible—breathe in the pain as you would hot, heavy air. Let go of any sense of blame or judgment. Breathe in the raw feeling directly as the hot, heavy air of pain. Take it in completely through every pore of your body. Own the rawness of it completely. This practice takes a lot of courage. You might find yourself resisting breathing in pain. You can breathe in anxiety, confusion, grief or frustration—whatever form your pain or suffering takes. Let the heart warm and beat as the steel sheath dissolves to reveal your spacious heart. Breathe out the sense of spaciousness, openness, kindness and surrender. When you breathe out, radiate positive energy completely, through all the pores of your body. Don't analyze what you are doing. Don't try to figure it out. Don't justify it. Simply do the practice. Breathe in the hot, heavy air of pain and breathe out a sense of spaciousness, openness, kindness and surrender. As you breathe in pain, own it completely. Then breathe out clarity, surrender and kindness. Take the time to lengthen and deepen each breath as you practice for a few minutes. End this practice by acknowledging your struggles and be kind to yourself. Notice what happens next.

Connecting with Those Who are Suffering

Now consider that at this very moment many others are experiencing a similar kind of pain as you. Being human means having pain. You don't have to imagine a particular person, although you may decide to dedicate this practice to a friend who also lives with pain or a group of people who have a similar condition. The point is to connect with the sensation that others are suffering just as you are. Feeling your distress and their distress, breathe it in for others as well as for yourself. Breathe this collective pain in as hot, heavy air. This won't increase your pain; rather, it will open your heart to the truth that, like you, all humans suffer. It will give you the opportunity to connect with them. Let this connectedness radiate compassion toward yourself and them. As you breathe out clarity, surrender, and kindness, let the breath go to all those who are suffering as you are. Take the time to lengthen and deepen each breath. Now dissolve the visualization and continue with the practice, breathing in universal suffering—your suffering and that of all humans—as heavy, hot air. The hardness around your heart dissolves, and your heart appears. End this practice acknowledging the suffering we share as humans and know you are not alone. Notice what happens next.

Tonglen is one of the bravest practices that a person can do. It dissolves the layers of self-protection we've tried so hard to create. It is a practice of great kindness that opens up our whole heart to the overwhelming presence of suffering and our strength and willingness to be with this openly. As you do this practice, gradually at your own pace, you will be surprised to find yourself more and more able to open up to your own pain. You will also build the resilience that is essential to living life fully and vibrantly. It can also help you to be there for others, even in situations that at one time may have seemed impossible.

PART V

Take Action and Do What Matters: Commit to a New and Vital Life Course

"In your pain you find your values, and in your values you find your pain"
– Steven C. Hayes

CHAPTER 29: BECOMING ACTIVE

Humans can take action even when the outcomes seem remote or unknown. A life lived according to values is described as rewarding, meaningful, fulfilling, active and deep. It can also feel liberating, joyous and free. For some, it is crystal clear why values are important. Although living by your values can be extremely rewarding, it is not always about living stress-free, being happy all the time, or even being pain-free.

If you look back on your own life, there may be clues about what it means to live by your values. If you think back on your life, you may realize that things that were important to you may have involved some kind of pain or suffering. For example: Each time you make a new friend, you risk social rejection. Every time you take on a new job you care about, you open yourself up to failure or criticism. Each time you exercise to feel and look better, you might experience some soreness and discomfort. Pain and values are poured from the same mold. What have you learned from your struggles?

Just thinking about values can cause suffering. You might become aware of what you have missed out on and how far you are from the kind of person you want to be or from the life you want to live. Just thinking about who and what you care about can be an emotional experience. If you notice strong emotions show up while exploring your values, it a sign that you are on the heels of something that's truly important to you.

There are no right or wrong values. Different people have different values, and no two people have the same mix. At different points in life some values carry more weight than others. If you have welcomed your first child into the world, your value of being a loving parent may overshadow all other values. Yet, those other values are still present—like being a supportive spouse and a community leader who helps those who are less fortunate. They just hold less attention in the moment.

We live in a very goal-oriented society and values are often confused with goals. Think of values as the direction you travel and goals as the destination you want to reach. Goals can be checked off a list, completed or achieved. Losing ten pounds is a goal; eating foods that nurture your health is a value. Getting married is a goal; being a loving and supportive spouse is a value. Winning the race to be town mayor is a goal; supporting members of the community is a value.

Values are like a compass. We use them to choose the direction in which we want to move and to help keep us on track as we travel. Values are like heading west. No matter how fast you travel you never get there; there is always further to go. But goals are the specific destinations you want to reach on your journey—they are like the sites you want to see or the mountains you want to climb while you travel west.

Values power our lives and empower us personally because they are always available to us. Your values guide the journey of your life. It can be useful to look back on an important time in your life in order to identify what values were behind your decisions. Embedded in these moments are the values that helped steer your life. There are many ways you can go about identifying your personally held values and this next exercise will help you do just that.

80th Birthday Celebration

Imagine you are attending your 80th birthday party. On this important day all of your closest friends, family and colleagues are at your party, ready to celebrate you and your life. Take a moment to think about who you really hope would be there. Think about friends, family members, co-workers and members of the community.

Before you light the cake and blow out the candles, one of your friends chooses to stand up and speak about you and the impact you have had on their life. This is their special way to honor you, the choices you have made in your life, what was important to you, and what you mean to them. One by one, each attendee stands and takes the microphone. Now imagine, what would you want them to say about you as a person? What would you want them to say about your role as a spouse, parent or sibling? How about as a co-worker or member of the community? Imagine what you would want them to say about the impact you've made and how you cared for and nurtured others or yourself? There might be memories shared of times when you acted in a loving way, or when you connected with others, or made a contribution to the community. Memories might be shared of times when you worked toward something important to you, courageous moments when you took bold action, or ways in which you lived life deliberately and purposefully.

Use the lines below to write down a few things you would want your loved ones to say about you.

_____
_____
_____
_____
_____
_____
_____
_____
_____
_____

Let that scene dissolve in your mind.

Now, try to imagine a different scenario. Imagine that it's your 80th birthday but you haven't lived a life based on your values and what's important to you. Instead, you were guided by the desire to avoid stress, by trying not to have unwanted thoughts, emotions or bodily sensations, while trying to control pain at all costs. From this different perspective, now that you have lived a long life, what would you fear has made up your life, if you did not act on your values?

After imagining a life of purpose and meaning versus a life ruled by fear and pain, what would your choices be now? What values would guide your choices and actions? What would you do differently? Each of us has only have a brief amount of time on this planet. Deep in your heart, what do you want your life to be about?

CHAPTER 30: CHOOSING A VALUE

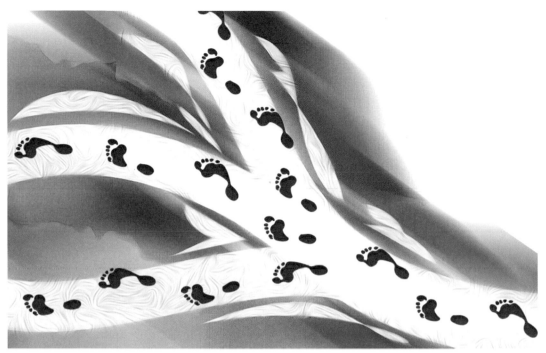

Reconnecting to your values can help you choose a path and move toward the life you desire.

When pain—or the fear of an activity that may cause pain—shows up, you likely respond by trying to reduce it, eliminate it, control it or distract from it. Your behavior changes in response to pain; this includes your thoughts, feelings and actions. Living life by your values requires action. Although it may not always feel like it, you have control over how you respond to pain when it shows up. Learning to take action and respond differently is the key to getting unstuck and living your values.

It is time to take a giant step, stride or leap forward toward the life you want. It is time to start walking in a direction toward life instead of away from who and what you care about. The journey of a thousand miles begins with just one step. This exercise will help you choose one value and put it in motion.

Ten Steps to Trying on a Value

Choose a value

- Choose a value you are willing to try on for at least a week. This should be a value that you care about and that you can realistically incorporate into your life. Below is a guide including common values that many people find important. Use this list to help you identify and clarify what is truly important to you. This list is by no means exhaustive, so feel free to add your own values.

• Accomplishment	• Fairness	• Kindness	• Rituals
• Action	• Faithfulness	• Laughter	• Sacredness
• Adventure	• Family	• Leadership	• Safety
• Appreciation	• Feelings	• Learning	• Security
• Attention	• Freedom	• Love	• Self-control
• Beauty	• Friendship	• Loyalty	• Self-expression
• Belief	• Fun	• Mastery	• Self-respect
• Calm	• Grace	• Nature	• Sensuality
• Challenge	• Gratitude	• Nurture	• Serenity
• Change	• Growth	• Openness	• Service
• Community	• Happiness	• Order	• Sexuality
• Compassion	• Health	• Parenting	• Spirituality
• Connection	• Home	• Partnership	• Spontaneity
• Consistency	• Honesty	• Passion	• Strength
• Contribution	• Honor	• Patience	• Structure
• Control	• Hope	• Peace	• Support
• Courage	• Humor	• Persuasion	• Surrender
• Creativity	• Imagination	• Planning	• Tradition
• Curiosity	• Independence	• Play	• Trust
• Dependability	• Inner Strength	• Pleasure	• Truth
• Dignity	• Inspiration	• Power	• Understanding
• Discovery	• Integrity	• Pride	• Vitality
• Empathy	• Intellect	• Quiet Admiration	• Wealth
• Encouragement	• Intuition	• Relationship	• Wholeness
• Enlightenment	• Invention	• Reliability	• Winning
• Equanimity	• Joy	• Respect	• Work
• Excellence	• Justice	• Risk	

Notice thoughts

- Notice any thoughts that come up about whether this value is good enough, or whether or not you really care about this value. Just notice all thoughts for what they are. Remember that your mind's job is to create thoughts. Let your mind do that as you continue with this exercise.

Make a list

- Take a moment to list a few behaviors that are related to the chosen value. For example: Connection with others, independence in making decisions, caring and nurturing health by attending a yoga class, cultivating ongoing and deep relationships by going to my parent's house for dinner.

Choose a behavior

- From this list, choose one behavior or set of behaviors you can commit to for at least a week.

Notice judgments

- Notice any feelings that come up about whether or not the behavior you've chosen to commit to is a good behavior, whether or not it will be pleasant or distressing, or whether you can actually do that to which you are committing yourself.

Make a plan

- Write down how you will go about incorporating this value in the very near future (today, tomorrow, this coming weekend, at the next meeting with your supervisor). Consider anything you will need to plan or get in order (e.g., call another person, clean the house, make an appointment, etc.). Choose when you will take this action—the sooner the better.

- *For example: I will connect with my best friend twice this week over lunch and listen intently as she speaks about her struggles, wants and joys or I will attend two 60-minute gentle yoga classes, or I will have dinner with my parents and express one sentiment of gratitude for our time spent together.*

Just act

- Even if this value involves other people, do not tell them what you are doing. See what you notice if you act on this value without talking to anyone about it.

Keep a daily diary of your reactions

- Pay attention to other's reactions to you and to any thoughts, feelings and body sensations that occur before, during and after you take action. Also, note how you feel when you act on this value for the second (or fifth, or tenth, or hundredth) time. Watch for thoughts that indicate whether this activity, value, or valued direction was "good" or "bad." Also, pay attention to judgments about yourself and others in relation to living this value. Thank your mind for those thoughts and see if you can choose not to buy into the judgments your mind makes about the activity.

Commit

- Commit to taking action in line with your values every day and notice anything that shows up as you do so.

Reflect

- After you have taken this action for a week, read through your daily reactions diary and reflect on what you have noticed and what you have learned.

CHAPTER 31: TAKING ACTION

In previous chapters, you learned how to make room for painful sensations in service of the way you want to live. You learned that your thoughts and feelings do not have to steer your life and you learned how to watch and defuse from them. You learned that letting go of pain control frees you to explore a new world full of possibilities. You also learned how to use your values to shape and mold your life rather than letting pain take the wheel.

When you merge a willingness to be with unpleasant inner experiences with the commitment to live life, true energy is generated to catapult life forward. From this perspective, you begin to see what you have control over. Along with your newfound willingness and commitment, there is still action to be taken.

The following exercise will help you choose and commit to an activity, identify how this action will move you closer to your goals and values, and identify the avoidance behaviors that will likely arise. You will also identify and be aware of the thoughts, feelings and sensations you're willing to make room for in order to achieve your goal. Fill in each box with as much information as possible and be specific in each area.

 Choose an Activity

Example: What is the activity I am committed to take? I will walk the dog for 30 minutes after my morning coffee.	**What is the activity I am committed to take?**
Example: How will this move me toward my values and goals? My goal is to walk for exercise 4 times per week for 30 minutes as a way to strengthen my knees because I value my health, wellbeing and the playful relationship I have with my grandchildren	**How will this move me toward my values and goals?**
Example: What avoidance behaviors am I willing to suspend in service of my value and goals? I will not make a second cup of coffee in the morning, sit on the couch, check Facebook or watch morning talk shows.	**What avoidance behaviors am I willing to suspend in service of my value and goals?**
Example: What unpleasant thoughts, emotions and sensations am I willing to make room for when completing the activity? I'm willing to make room for some knee pain and feeling hot and sweaty. I also notice that I'm having thoughts that too much exercise will damage my knees and I'm going to have to use a walker for the rest of my live. I'm willing to move and walk with these thoughts because I value my health and family.	**What unpleasant thoughts, emotions and sensations am I willing to make room for when completing the activity?**

CHAPTER 32: LIFE IN THE BULLSEYE

Throughout this book, you've completed exercises to help you discover who and what is most important in your life. You've rediscovered old values, identified new ones, and clarified what is most meaningful—the activities that bring you wellbeing and vitality.

Now that you have identified some of your values, the next step on the journey is to consider where you are in relation to each of these values. In other words, are you living in accordance with your values? Are you doing the things you've identified as important and meaningful? Living your values isn't a goal; it isn't a destination that you arrive at one day, making it complete. Living your values involves a series of actions you continually take and an ongoing process you live every day for the rest of your life. Values aren't a destination; they are your north star and guiding light. What will you do today to live life in line with your values?

Take a moment to reflect on how you have behaved over the last few weeks or month. Were your actions and behavior consistent with your values? Did they reflect the person you want to be? The next exercise will help you identify if your behavior is supporting your values so that you can take action each day and begin to live in line with your valued choices.

The Bullseye is an exercise that is divided into four important areas of living: work, love, play and health.

Work includes your job and career aims. For those not working, this may apply to school or volunteer activities. Do you work, study or do another meaningful activity in this area? How do you want to treat your clients, customers, colleagues, employees and fellow workers? What personal qualities do you want to bring to your work? What skills do you want to develop? What further training would you like to pursue? This includes your values about career advancement, further training, education or knowledge.

Play includes your leisure activities. How do you play, relax, or enjoy yourself during your free time? What are your hobbies or other activities for rest, recreation, fun and creativity? Some hobbies or activities could include gardening, sewing, bird watching, travel, coaching a children's sports team, fishing, playing sports, etc.

Love includes the meaningful social connections in your life, including relationships with your children, parents, siblings, spouse or partner, your friends, and acquaintances in the community. Which relationships do you want to build and cultivate? How do you want to be in these relationships? What personal qualities do you want to develop?

Health includes five important areas including physical activity, nutrition, sleep, buffering stress, and reflecting on risk factors related to wellbeing—such as drinking, drug use, smoking and maintaining a healthy weight.

With the Bullseye exercise, you will look more closely at your personal values in each of these areas and write them down. Then, you will evaluate how close you are to living your life in line with your values. You will also take a closer look at the barriers or obstacles in your life that stand between you and the kind of life you want to live. Set aside some quiet time to dedicate to this exercise.

Identify Your Values

Start by describing your values within each of the four areas of living as described on the previous page. Think about each area in terms of your dreams, imagining the possibility of having your wishes completely fulfilled. What are the qualities that you would like to get out of each area and what are your expectations from these areas of your life? Your values should not be specific goals but instead reflect a way you would like to live your life over time. For example, getting married might be a goal you have in life, and it reflects the value of being an affectionate, honest and loving partner. To accompany your daughter to a softball game might be a goal; to be an involved and interested parent might be the value. Write your values for each area on the lines provided below. It is your personal values that are important in this exercise.

Work:

_____

_____

Play:

_____

_____

Love:

_____

_____

Health:

_____

_____

Now, look again at the values you have written above. Think of your value as a "Bullseye" (the center of the dartboard). Being in the center of the Bullseye is exactly where you want to be—living your life in a way that is consistent with your values. You have hit the mark! Place an X on the dartboard in each area that best represents where you stand today. An X in the center of the Bullseye means that you are living completely in keeping with your value for that area of living. An X on the outside and far from the center of the Bullseye means that your life is way off the mark in terms of how you are living your life. Since there are four areas of valued living, you should mark four X's on the dartboard.

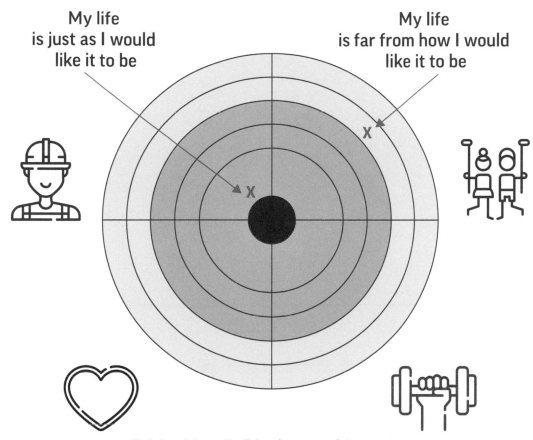

My life
is just as I would
like it to be

My life
is far from how I would
like it to be

X

X

The Bullseye helps you identify how close you are to living your values.

Take Valued Action

Think about actions you can take in your daily life to help you get closer to the Bullseye in each important area of your life. These actions could be small steps toward a particular goal, or they could be actions that reflect what you want to be about as a person. Usually, taking a valued step includes being willing to encounter the obstacles you identified earlier and to take the action anyway. Try to identify at least one value-based action you are willing to take in each of the four areas listed below.

Work:

_____

_____

Play:

_____

_____

Love:

_____

_____

Health:

_____

_____

Identify Your Obstacles

Now write down what stands between you and living your life as you want to, from what you have written in your areas of value on page 88. When you think of the life you want to live and the values that you would like to put in play, what gets in the way of you living that kind of life? Also, estimate to what extent the obstacles can prevent you from living your life in a way that is in keeping with your values. Place a number next to the obstacle that best describes how powerful this obstacle is in your life. 1 = Doesn't prevent me at all, 5 = Prevents me completely

Describe any obstacle(s) on the lines below.

Obstacle(s) to living your values at work:

_____

_____1 2 3 4 5

Obstacle(s) to living your values at play:

_____

_____1 2 3 4 5

Obstacle(s) to living your values in love:

_____

_____1 2 3 4 5

Obstacle(s) to living your values in health:

_____

_____1 2 3 4 5

The aim of the Bullseye exercise is to build awareness around the activities that make you feel vital, as well as the choices and actions you can take each day to keep your life moving in the right direction. It is natural that one of the four areas is far away from the center, while others may be closer to hitting the mark. This is to be expected. It is also normal that as you move through different parts of your life and your values change, your location on the Bullseye will change as well. Some days you may be very close in all areas, and other days you may be far away. The Bullseye isn't a measure to judge your performance but a guide, similar to the compass that you can use to help you continually move in the desired direction for your values. Whether you are taking big steps or small steps, as long as you are moving along with your values you are on the right path. Your greatest successes are achieved when moving in direction with your values.

CHAPTER 33: DIALING UP WILLINGNESS

There is no pain switch that we can flip on and off. Nor is there a switch for our thoughts, feelings and bodily sensations. By now you understand that even if there were such a switch, there would be ramifications for such an intervention. Still, we hope for such a breakthrough and try things without success. A client of mine, named Judy, had her own experience with solutions that promised to switch pain off.

Judy was a very active woman, married, with two kids in high school. She ran a boutique children's clothing store well known by many in the community. Her friends and family knew Judy as full of energy, able to manage the complexities of running a business, caring for a family and nurturing her own health. Judy did it all, including playing tennis four times a week at the local club until a back injury took her out of the game. Not only was she not able to play tennis anymore, but Judy was laid out flat on her back for months, unable to work or care for her family. During this time, she had to turn the management of her business over to someone. She no longer was there to prep her kids' lunch in the morning, pick them up for school, or attend their extracurricular activities. Her relationship with her friends was practically non-existent, her husband was tired of her complaints of pain and he missed her as a life partner. She tried many of the conservative measures that are common, including physical therapy, massage, chiropractic care, relaxation therapy, over the counter pain killers, and even a steroid injection. No relief was to be found. After many months of suffering, Judy reluctantly agreed to the surgeon's suggestion that back surgery was the only way out. She went under the knife and a portion of the problematic disc was removed. Unfortunately for Judy, the surgery was a failure. Not only did it fail to provide pain relief but she now relied on a strong narcotic opioid.

When I first saw Judy, she was desperate and depressed and wanted nothing more than to come off the narcotic painkiller but reported that she needed it. She reported it helped her 7/10 pain, and it helped ease her mounting anxiety over losing her job, her deteriorating finances, her difficult home life and absence of close, personal relationships. As many painkillers do, it worked for a short period of time, for a few hours each day, but it mostly left her passed out asleep on the living room couch. Judy ran through all the options of available pain management and was at the end of her rope. As a last-ditch effort, Judy was referred to me for pain exposure therapy. This special type of treatment helps you face your fears about pain, movement and activity. It can be used for any sort of anxiety but is often used to break the cycle of pain by tackling fear and avoidance, which often accompanies chronic pain.

During our earliest treatment sessions, we worked together on breathing, being with the pain in the moment, and not letting it pull her into past thoughts or future fears. Then we moved to observing all the content of the mind that came with pain—the thoughts, feelings and emotions that were caked on and layered on top of pain. Then we practiced being with different bodily sensations that were unpleasant like breathing heavy, a racing pulse, pounding heartbeat, muscles contracting and sweaty palms. Finally, exercises to open up to some pain while she moved her spine and body in all different directions, many of them that were similar to the daily activities she once pursued before pain. At first, none of this was very pleasant for Judy, and some days hurt more than others. Some exercises were scary and caused some anxiety. As Judy stayed with the treatment she reported being able to do more, return to some of the things she cared about, and was less focused on pain.

One day, Judy showed up to therapy with what she called an *aha* moment, which she described: "On my way to therapy this morning I was thinking that I've lost a whole year of my life. I've lost money because I can't work, and my store is a mess without me. I don't see my friends anymore or play tennis and my physical health has suffered. My family thinks I've all but checked out and turned into a drug addict. My husband is sick of hearing about my pain and our relationship is on the last straw. For the past year I've been looking for ways to decrease pain. I've seen everyone and tried everything. None of it has really worked and most of the solutions people have recommended have only made things worse. This time and your exercises have taught me that I'm focusing in the wrong place. So many of my waking hours are dedicated to fighting pain that I have no time or energy left for anything else. Along the way I've learned that I'm stronger than I thought and can handle some things that hurt and still do what I want. I'm ready to go back to work and take responsibility for the house and kids again. I know it may hurt some days and it will take a long time for my pain to go away. Heck, I'm not even sure it will ever go away! But I'm also seeing everything I care about slipping away—especially my husband and my children, whom I cherish. I'm willing to work with what I have today if it means getting my life and family back again!"

Judy had reached an invisible boundary she was ready to cross over. She acknowledged that she cannot change pain. Her own life experience coupled with the exposure therapy built courage so she could change the things she could, and she developed wisdom to see that pain was running her life.

Each day presents opportunities for us to open up to pain if it is in service of the things we love and follow in life rather than following relief. There is no pain switch we can flip on and off, but we can adjust our level of willingness. We learn to embrace unpleasant events. We let our thoughts and emotions just be as they are, not as we would have them. All types of bodily sensations buzz in the background. When you come in contact with pain you can adjust your willingness dial. Instead of shutting off pain, you dial up willingness.

 ## The Willingness Dial

Below are two dials. One dial for willingness and another dial for pain. Set the dial to your current pain level. Most people living with pain have their willingness dial set to 0 and their pain dial set very high. Below is a picture of what struggling with pain looks like on these two dials.

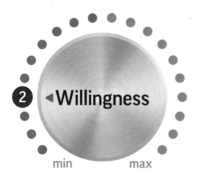

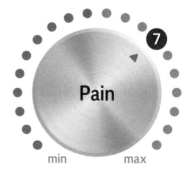

We have almost no control over the pain dial. The willingness dial can be ratcheted up or down as life requires. Judy learned to adjust her willingness dial when it mattered most, during times with her family and work. During the important moments in her life the dials looked like the ones below:

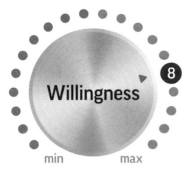 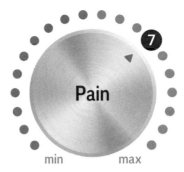

Here is a table showing how Judy's adjusted willingness dial changed with different activities in her life. Notice that with some activities Judy turned up the willingness dial to its maximum. These were activities that were important and meaningful to her, yet she feared them—like activity #3—Judy was scared of how golf would affect her back. With other activities—such as #1 (returning to work) she did not have to dial up willingness as much.

Activity #1 Returning to work 3 days per week for 7 hours each day in her store.	Willingness 8 — Pain 7
Activity #2 Make breakfast, prepare lunch, and make sure her children catch the bus in the morning.	Willingness 9 — Pain 7
Activity #3 Nine holes of golf on Sunday and lunch date after with her husband.	Willingness 10 — Pain 7
Activity #4 Dinner and book club with friends.	Willingness 7 — Pain 7

Using the table below, choose five activities that are important to you and set your willingness dial accordingly for each activity. These should be activities you have avoided or partially avoided since living with pain. These do not have to be the most challenging activities or ones that cause you the most distress, but they should be important ones.

As you write down the activities below, remember that I am not asking you to tolerate pain, resign to it or give in. Tolerating pain or giving in is the mind's way of avoiding. Willingness is visible: your body can be observed doing something new or different. Depending on the activity, you can turn the willingness dial up for a specific amount of time, such as going to a movie for two hours. Once that activity is complete you can turn the willingness dial back down as you return home and rest. Try and set your willingness dial to at least a seven for each activity. This demonstrates that you are ready to allow (feel) unpleasant sensations in order to do something of value.

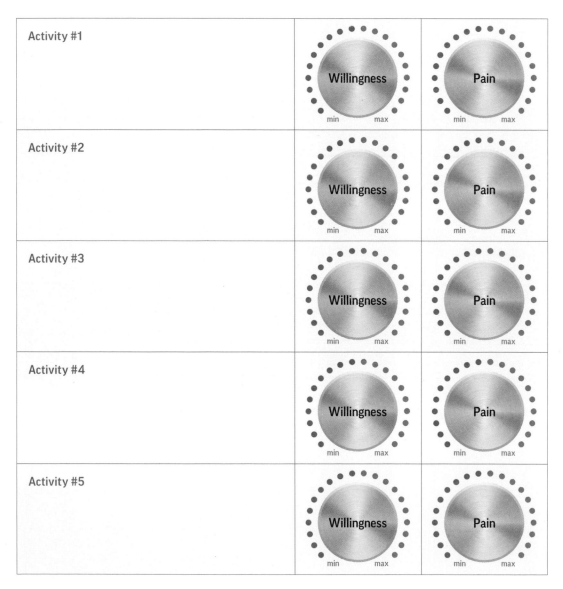

How would you handle your life differently if you were focused on adjusting your willingness dial? For today, turn up the willingness dial and act in a way that increases your quality of life.

CHAPTER 34: NAVIGATING THE PATH

Valued living involves discovering what we want out of life and then making a commitment to ourselves to take action in service of those values. Essentially, it is the most vital way we could choose to live.

Values guide us on our chosen paths as we define what is important and meaningful. A life driven by values is a fully vital life characterized by wholeness, fullness, purpose, some pleasure and some discomfort and pain. Even if you are in close contact with your values, your mind can pull you away from what is meaningful by setting the traps of obstacles along your path. These obstacles are the inner experiences that cause us to struggle. When we believe thoughts are real, we are pulled back into avoidance, creating distance from our values. If we put off valued living until the uncomfortable thoughts, feelings and sensations "go away," or are "fixed," the path becomes overgrown and we can't see the forest for the trees.

This process can be compared with taking a hike in the mountains. The mountain is tall and steep, and switchbacks require you to walk back and forth on the winding trail. At certain points, the trail drops back below a level you had reached earlier. If I asked you to evaluate how well you were accomplishing your goal of reaching the mountaintop, I would hear a different story depending on where you were on the trail. If you were on a switchback, you would probably tell me that things weren't going well, that you were never going to reach the top. If you were on a stretch of open trail, where you could see the mountaintop and the path leading up to it, you would probably tell me things were going great. Now, imagine being across the valley with a pair of binoculars, watching other people hiking on this trail. If we asked how they were doing, it would be a positive progress report every time. We would be able to see that the overall direction of the trail (not what it looks like at a given moment) is the key to progress. We would see that this crazy, winding trail leads to the top.

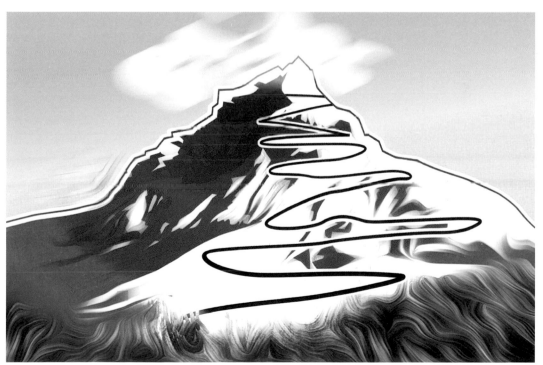

The path toward your values may wind back and forth but it ultimately leads to the mountaintop.

Overcoming pain can be like scaling a mountain. Sometimes it's sunny and clear, and at other times a cloud rolls in and covers the summit. Sometimes the path is well-worn with places to securely place your feet as you ascend, and at other times you're treading on loose gravel and have to be careful not to slip and sprain an ankle. The best hikers have an important navigation tool to help them find their way: a compass. It needs no batteries and can be used with or without a map.

A compass gives you a direction to follow, keeps you on track and prevents you from getting lost. Values are your compass; they help create a path as you journey through life. Values are what we find meaningful in life. They are what you deeply care about and consider to be important. Values are different for everybody, and may change over time, depending on the season of your life.

Values are different from goals, which can be written on a list and checked off. Values are more like a compass direction that you want to head in. When you act on a value, it's like heading west, or heading toward the sunset. No matter how far west you travel, you never get there and there's always further to go. You never reach the sunset, but you continue to move towards it. Goals are different, They are like the achievements you want to make on your journey—the sights you want to see or the mountains you want to climb. For example, you might have the goal of getting to work on time, with the value of being a good employee, or the goal of completing a 5k race, while placing value on regular exercise and physical health.

Even if you learn to enjoy a challenge and tend to push your body to new limits, which can feel great, you may encounter your fair share of problems along the way. You might experience foot pain or knee pain, or your mind might start telling you to turn back or take another path. The values compass will keep you going. As long as you keep moving in the direction of your values, it will always point you toward the brilliant beauty of lavender sunsets, making the journey worth it!

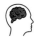 ## Life Compass

The categories on the chart are key areas that are valued by most people. Setting aside any obstacles for the moment, think about what is important to you, and what you think makes for a meaningful life guided by values. For each category, write one sentence summarizing a value you hold dear. For example, "to live a healthy life and nurture my body" (Physical Wellbeing) or, "to be a loving and caring wife" (Marriage). You can come back to the compass and review these phrases should you find yourself pulled off the path. A few examples are provided below to help you.

Being a supportive and loving wife.

Being a deeply caring and loving parent.

A team player at work.

A leader in my community.

A leader in my profession.

A shoulder for those in need.

Living life as a good Christian/Jew/Muslim/Buddhist.

Nurturing and caring for my body.

The creative process of making new music that brings people joy.

Care for my son to see him through his battle with depression.

Treat my body like a sacred temple.

A constant quest for self-improvement.

Learning new things.

Rehabilitating my body so I can care for my family.

To strengthen my body by eating well and getting plenty of exercise and sleep.

To live a life free of medications.

To feel loved and accepted for who I am.

To be someone who helps vulnerable children.

To be someone who is in touch with nature.

Someone always deepening their spiritual journey.

To pursue and explore my creative talents.

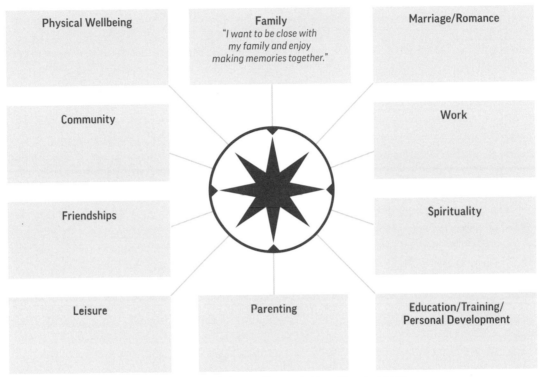

Physical Wellbeing

Family
"I want to be close with my family and enjoy making memories together."

Marriage/Romance

Community

Work

Friendships

Spirituality

Leisure

Parenting

Education/Training/ Personal Development

The life compass can help you rediscover what is most important to you.

This activity gives you the opportunity to investigate and discover what you want your life to be about. Up until now, it's likely that pain has defined your life and kept you locked horns in a struggle. I doubt that's what you want. Calibrating your compass is one way to reclaim your life from pain. Although this approach may seem backward, it truly is the way forward. This is the great paradox of pain, and it brings you one step closer to Radical Relief. You are learning to dive into the wave instead of turning and running from it. Living life fully in the 10 valued areas above creates an environment that's hard for pain to thrive for very long. Wouldn't it be more fulfilling to live your life by your values, rather than to live it ruled by pain?

Still, there may be some pain. By now, you are beginning to see that some days the storm clouds roll in over the mountaintop. It showers you with rain, drenches your boots and chills you to the bone. On those days, consider whether trying to control or battle pain is really worth sacrificing all the areas that you've identified as meaningful and important. Remember the people, places and things you most care about reside in those values. May this give you hope, inspiration and vitality to live in service of what you truly value.

CHAPTER 35: REDISCOVER WHAT'S IMPORTANT

Values are the missing ingredient in the secret sauce to overcoming pain. They are rarely talked about and most people simply breeze right over them, forget about or ignore them. However, if there was one way to help you out of the pit of despair that pain sucked you into, it's your values. Let's take a deeper dive and explore ten key areas where values play an important role. There are many more, but this list will provide you with a solid foundation to rediscover who and what is most important in your life. One aspect of quality of life involves the importance you put on different areas of living. This questionnaire will help clarify your quality of life in each of these areas.

Rate the importance of each area (by circling a number) on a scale of 1-10. A "1" means that area is not at all important. A "10" means that area is very important to you. Not everyone will value all areas the same. It's okay to have several values scoring the same number. I encourage you to think about your entire life, including before you experienced pain, as you choose a score. Rate each area according to your own personal sense of importance. We also ask you to describe each area. Take note not to describe it since pain has entered your life. Describe it as you would have when you were feeling your best. Write a brief summary, in one or two sentences, or a few key words. I've provided some examples to help guide you.

Explore Your Unique Values

1) Family

	Not Important					Very Important			
1	2	3	4	5	6	7	8	9	10

This area describes the relationships you have with members of your family including parents, siblings, grandparents, cousins and other members of your extended family. What would you like these relationships to be about? Describe the qualities of these relationships as you would like them to be. What sort of brother/sister, son/daughter, uncle/aunt do you want to be? What personal qualities would you like to bring to these relationships? What sort of relationships would you like to build? How would you interact with others if you were the ideal you in these relationships?

_____

_____

_____

_____

2) Marriage/Romance

	Not Important					Very Important			
1	2	3	4	5	6	7	8	9	10

This area describes your relationship with your spouse, partner, boyfriend, girlfriend or that special someone in your life. What sort of partner would you like to be in an intimate relationship? What personal qualities would you like to develop? What sort of relationship would you like to build? How would you interact with your partner if you were the "ideal you" in this relationship?

_____

_____

_____

_____

3) Parenting
Not Important   Very Important
1 2 3 4 5 6 7 8 9 10

This area describes what sort of parent you would like to be. What sort of qualities would you like to have? What sort of relationships would you like to build and nurture with your children as they grow and age? How would you behave if you were the "ideal" you?

_____
_____
_____
_____

4) Friendships
Not Important   Very Important
1 2 3 4 5 6 7 8 9 10

This area describes your social life. What qualities would you like to bring to your friendships and social circles? If you could be the best friend possible, how would you behave towards your friends? What sort of friendships would you like to build?

_____
_____
_____
_____

5) Work/Career
Not Important   Very Important
1 2 3 4 5 6 7 8 9 10

This area describes what you value in your work. What would make it more meaningful? What kind of worker would you like to be? What kind of co-worker would you like to be? If you were living up to your own ideal standards, what personal qualities would you like to bring to your work or team? What sort of work relationships would you like to build?

_____
_____
_____
_____

6) Education/Training/Personal Development
Not Important   Very Important
1 2 3 4 5 6 7 8 9 10

This area encompasses education, training, personal growth and development. What do you value about learning, education, training or personal growth? What new skills would you like to learn? What knowledge would you like to gain? What further education appeals to you? What sort of student would you like to be? What personal qualities would you like to apply?

_____
_____
_____
_____

7) Recreation & Hobbies

Not Important					Very Important				
1	2	3	4	5	6	7	8	9	10

This area describes all the areas where you seek out fun and entertainment. What sorts of hobbies, sports, or leisure activities do you enjoy? How do you relax and unwind? How do you have fun? What sorts of activities would you like to do?

_____

_____

_____

8) Spirituality

Not Important					Very Important				
1	2	3	4	5	6	7	8	9	10

Whatever spirituality means to you is fine. This could be religion or a spiritual practice. It may be as simple as communing with nature, or as formal as participation in an organized religious group, church, synagogue or mosque. What is important to you in this area of life?

_____

_____

_____

9) Community/Citizenship

Not Important					Very Important				
1	2	3	4	5	6	7	8	9	10

This area describes how you would like to contribute to your community or environment. This could be through volunteering, supporting a group, working with a charity or a political party. What sort of environments would you like to create at home, work or in the spaces you live? What environments would you like to spend more time in?

_____

_____

_____

10) Health & Wellness

Not Important					Very Important				
1	2	3	4	5	6	7	8	9	10

This area encompasses your physical and mental health. What are your values related to maintaining your well-being? How do you want to look after your health, with regard to sleep, diet, exercise, smoking, alcohol, etc.? Why is this important?

_____

_____

_____

Look back now and circle the areas that are most important to you. Also, note if there any areas that surprised you. Are there areas you are ready to reconnect with or explore? Values are what help you live a rich, meaningful and active life even when complete pain relief is not possible. The interesting thing about values is they are unique to you and your life. No two people have the same mix of values. Guided by your personal and unique values, you are prepared to navigate these important areas of life.

CHAPTER 36: STAYING ON COURSE

During your struggle with pain, you've probably realized that certain unpleasant thoughts, feelings, sensations and memories can get in the way of the direction you want to go and the life you want to live. These are the things that keep you stuck. A great deal of this book has been dedicated to becoming more aware of these thoughts, feelings, sensations, and memories in the present moment. You also realize your deep and personally held values are what keep you moving in your chosen life direction. The next exercise, The Life Line, is designed to help you explore areas where you are stuck and what happens as a consequence. These are the areas where moving in a valued direction has become difficult due to obstacles or internal experiences.

 The Life Line

Step 1: Think of a current value that feels far away, remote or compromised due to some sort of barrier. Write the value in the box at the top of the Life Line arrow on page 102. Notice that there is distance between where you are today, standing at the beginning of the line, and the value you want to move toward.

Step 2: Close your eyes and imagine a special activity you enjoy. Make it an activity that you have not been able to return to doing or successfully engage with. This would be an activity that helps you move toward your values, and if you knew you could do it, you'd be stronger and healthier. Imagine you are doing the activity here and now and just experience what it feels like in your body (one minute). This is you moving along the Life Line toward your values.

Step 3: Now imagine someone is standing over you, criticizing you for not being able to do the activity, demanding achievement and results from this activity. Notice how that feels. This could be what the Protector Within says or what it urges you to do or not do in its attempts to keep you safe and protected from pain.

Step 4: Now notice any internal barriers that show up. A barrier can be defined as anything that gets in the way of living your values and achieving a rich, meaningful and active life. These can be identified in four areas which are unpleasant thoughts, feelings, sensations or memories. For each category, be specific and write down any internal barrier that shows up as you try and move toward your chosen value. Write these down on the left-hand side of the Life Line on page 102.

Step 5: When the barriers appear, and the unpleasant sensations show up, what type of **behaviors** do you engage in to control or avoid pain? Think long and hard about these, this can be a tricky area. It is common to only identify one avoidance behavior, but after reflecting longer you will probably notice that many exist. These include behaviors to decrease pain, avoid pain, distract, numb out, zone out, check out, feel good, soothe or calm. These are often identified as behaviors such as getting lost by watching TV, sleeping, not exercising, crying, fighting with a loved one, surfing the internet, drinking alcohol or overly relying on medication. Even seemingly *positive behaviors* such as reading, relaxation exercises or gentle stretching can be an avoidance activity if it prevents you from moving toward your life's goals or values. Write the avoidance behaviors in the boxes on the right side on page 102. These are the behaviors that keep you stuck in the loop of pain control and avoidance.

Step 6: Check to see if any patterns emerge, such as surfing the internet or distracting with activities to soothe or control pain. Notice if these avoidance strategies help you move forward along the Life Line or hook you and pull you off the Line and away from your values. Have these avoidance strategies worked for you in the long run? What have they cost you in terms of work, play, love or health? What is it like standing here with the awareness of these avoidance strategies as well as how far you are away from your value?

Step 7: Finally, with your eyes closed think about how you will respond differently to these internal barriers if they were to show up again. Notice and name the barrier and then choose how you will proceed along the path despite these barriers and not let yourself get tugged off the Life Line by avoidance and control. Name one thing you will do differently when these barriers place a roadblock in your path.

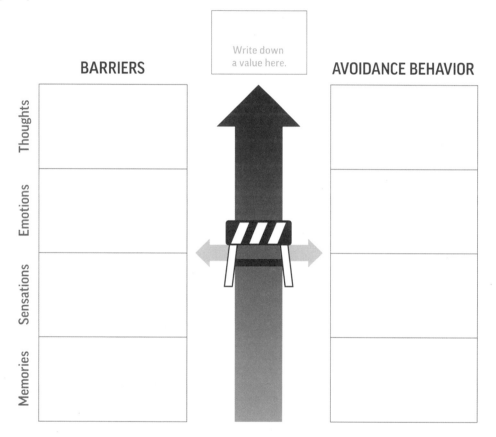

The Life Line exercise can be used for any number of your personally held values and the barriers that get in the way. It serves to show you which unpleasant internal experiences show up and prevent you from engaging with a full and active life. These are the barriers we do not so readily see because they are internal. Writing them down increases our awareness. On the right side are the behaviors you adopt or perform in the present moment to avoid feeling bad and willingly opening up to pain. The greater awareness you have of both the internal barriers and the avoidance strategies, the faster you can learn to be with them and not let them interfere with your life. Opening up to and willingly accepting unpleasant internal sensations and recognizing their presence in the moment will enable you to choose a different action. This can help you to do what is important to move steadily along the Life Line back to a full and active life.

CONCLUSION: MOVING TOWARD LIFE

All of us wish for a happy life free from pain and suffering. It is part of our human nature and evolutionary biology. Yet, life can get messy and emotions, habits and events will show up that may act as barriers to leading a rich, meaningful and active life. But this doesn't mean you have to suffer, live in fear or miss out on all that life has to offer.

Radical Relief does happen. You can live life without pain controlling you and without being caught in the traps and promises of pain relief. It doesn't mean that you'll never feel pain again and it doesn't mean you won't have thoughts that tell you to avoid pain. You will. To be human means you will experience pain, but it doesn't mean you have to suffer. The worst part of suffering is losing contact with who and what is important to you because pain has taken over.

Radical Relief entails noticing all that is unpleasant about pain and then choosing to respond differently. You can control how you respond. These are the seeds that cultivate radical change. You can learn to think, feel and experience old memories while still moving forward to create the life you desire. This is what makes up Radical Relief and the stance you can take each and every day. In cultivating this psychological flexibility, you are able to loosen your attachment to the fruitless struggle, and willingly work with the unchangeable with confidence and poise. You can also develop skills to engage more fully in meaningful and valued life activities, even in the presence of pain, stress and discomfort. Life becomes more about the people and activities that truly matter, and life satisfaction grows while pain takes up less space and consumes less mental and emotional energy.

If you advance confidently in the direction of your values, take some risks, and bravely dare to live the life which you have imagined while reading this book, you will meet with unexpected success. There will be obstacles to overcome. But as you leave the struggle with pain behind, you will pass an invisible boundary. The goal of this book is to help you reconstruct a solid foundation under your dreams. It is time to recognize that which can be changed and that which is out of your personal control and commit to taking action to enrich your life.

The rules and laws of pain as you knew them have changed. Pain is less complex now that you see that you are not broken, weak or damaged. You have learned how pain works and how to respond to your body and mind. It is time now to take one last brave stance and commit. For this last exercise, I invite you to stand up and finish the following sentences. You can also write these down and tape them to your mirror or make them into a screen saver on your computer or smartphone. Say them out loud in a confident voice, with your head held high. You've earned this through your dedication, and this is a powerful way to honor your work and achievements. These three phrases summarize an acceptance and mindful approach to living life.

Commitment to a New Way of Living

What I truly care about is _____.

What I've been doing is _____.
I'm through with that!

From today forward, I commit to _____.

You've created the conditions necessary to thrive in life, even if pain decides to arc back around. You are no longer stuck suffering—you now have tools to advance. You've learned to make room for and open up to pain guided by your values, which has allowed you to engage more fully with life. At the heart of this book and your new approach to life is the **MOVE** approach.

Make room for unpleasant sensations
Open-up and observe non-judgmentally
Values guide life, not pain
Engage in activities in line with your values

You can come back to this as a refresher, or whenever you feel stuck, require support or need a reminder.

Overcoming pain is no easy feat, but you are strong and resilient. As you complete this book, pain may have begun to reveal its purpose. It is natural for people who have found some respite from suffering to pay it forward and share what they have learned. Pain is a huge problem that affects billions of people around the world and a lot of work and healing is required. If you have benefited from the knowledge you learned in this book, you can be part of the solution. Research shows that when we help others, we help ourselves, which can alleviate suffering. If you feel called to help others overcome pain, I invite you to share this knowledge and help others find Radical Relief.

Go forward and share this knowledge with your friends, family and acquaintances. Start a book club or share this with your practitioner. The best way to continually practice and grow with this newfound knowledge is to teach others. In addition to living a life filled with meaning and purpose, driven by your most important values, sharing this knowledge is another profound way that pain can reveal a purpose. I wish you the best of luck and good health on the continuous journey to Radical Relief.

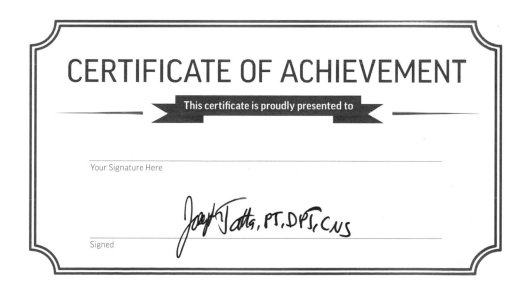

CERTIFICATE OF ACHIEVEMENT

This certificate is proudly presented to

_____
Your Signature Here

_____
Signed